Law on Poisons, Medicines and Related Substances

Studies in Law & Practice for Health Service Management (No.9)

Law on Poisons, Medicines and Related Substances

P. F. C. Bayliss,

LLB, MB, ChB, MRCP (Lond)

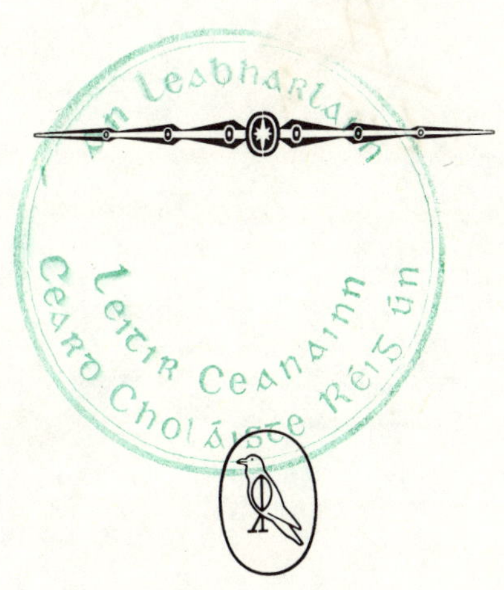

RAVENSWOOD PUBLICATIONS

P.O. Box No. 24, 205 Croydon Road, Beckenham, Kent, BR3 3AL, England

Published by
RAVENSWOOD PUBLICATIONS LTD
P.O. Box No. 24, 205 Croydon Road,
Beckenham, Kent, BR3 3AL, England

Published 1980

ISBN 0 901812 34 X soft cover
ISBN 0 901812 35 8 hard cover

Printed in Great Britain by
Biddles Ltd, Guildford, Surrey

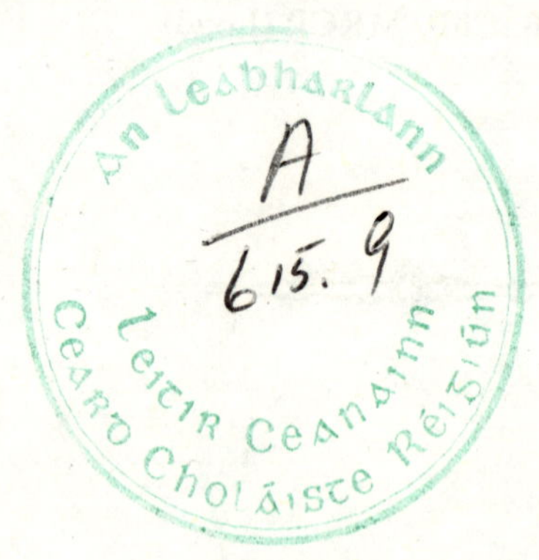

Contents

Preface

In 1968 a new comprehensive set of legal controls on medicinal products was introduced by the Medicines Act and the Regulations made under it. As this Act controlled many substances previously controlled under the Pharmacy and Poisons Act 1933 a new Act was introduced in 1972 to control non-medicinal poisons – The Poisons Act. At the same time the law on drugs of addiction was strengthened and consolidated in the Misuse of Drugs Act 1971. Anyone working in the Health Service, be they at a professional or administrative level, will require a working knowledge of these three statutes and the Body of Regulations made under them.

In this book Dr. Bayliss, who is qualified in medicine and law, and has worked both in the National Health Service and the pharmaceutical industry, gives an account of the legal controls on poisons, dangerous drugs and medicinal products. The historical background to this legislation is examined, and the last chapter presents a summary of other branches of the law that may have a bearing on this group of substances.

The book will be of value to anyone working in hospitals, nursing homes and in the Health Service and will be of particular interest to doctors, dentists, pharmacists, nurses, midwives and administrators.

Acknowledgments

I should like to thank Dr. W. A. J. Farndale, general editor of this series for his help and encouragement in writing this book; my colleagues Mr. F. G. Farrell B.Pharm., F.P.S., F.R.I.C. and Mr. B. Wienholt M.P.S. Barrister at Law, for reading the draft manuscript; and, as always, my wife for her constant support.

P. F. C. Bayliss

May, 1980

Table of Statutes

List of Statutory Instruments

Medicines Act 1968

Medicines Act 1968 (continued)

Medicines Act 1968 (continued)

Medicines Act 1968 (continued)

Misuse of Drugs Act 1971

The Misuse of Drugs –

Poisons Act 1972

List of Cases

Chapter One

Review of Legislation

It would be hard to imagine a building which houses a wider variety of dangerous substances than a hospital. Highly poisonous formalin and phenolic disinfectants. Deadly poison like strychnine. Powerful modern medicines that cure when used correctly but threaten life when used carelessly. Narcotics, like heroin and morphine, which are not only dangerous in their own right but addictive. Alcohol ranging from 'medicinal brandy' to methylated spirits. And radioactive substances which are used increasingly for diagnosis and treatment but which can present a whole range of new dangers.

Inevitably these and other substances have become subject to a large body of law devised to ensure through various controls and safeguards that their dangers are minimised or ideally eliminated entirely while at the same time allowing their undoubted benefits to be fully realised.

The law in this field has developed piecemeal and usually in response to specific problems.

The first relevant statute, the Arsenic Act 1851, was prompted by the use of the poison for murder and suicide. In the 1914-18 war controls were introduced under the Defence of the Realm (Consolidation) Regulations to combat cocaine addiction among the troops, and nearly 50 years later the Drugs (Prevention of Misuse) Act 1964 was implemented to deal with the widespread misuse of amphetamine in the early 1960s. The introduction of the Medicines Act in 1968, controlling the quality, safety and efficacy of medicinal products, arose partly from the thalidomide tragedy which highlighted the lack of statutory controls on the safety of new drugs.

Three Categories

The range of substances which are controlled in some way or another is extensive but three broad categories have emerged over the years – narcotic drugs, poisons and medicines. The law relating to these categories has recently been extended, consolidated and rationalised and is now contained in three modern statutes: the Misuse of Drugs Act 1971, the Poisons Act 1972 and the Medicines Act 1968.

Broad Problems Associated with Drugs and Poisons

The need for legal controls becomes apparent when considering the broad problems associated with narcotic drugs, poisons and modern medicines.

Addiction

One of the biggest problems concerns addiction. Some substances such as the narcotic drugs, morphine and pethidine, are valuable therapeutic agents. Others are of little or no value in therapy – LSD and marihuana for example, but all are capable of producing an overpowering desire to continue taking them. The tendency to increase the doses becomes stronger and stronger and mental and physical dependence occurs. The social consequences of addiction can be profound. They include disintegration of the personality and a tendency to dishonesty in order to obtain drug supplies or the money to buy them.

The addicts' craving for drugs has led to a world-wide network of illegal drug suppliers. In this context the hazard of the so-called 'soft' drugs – those which are only weakly addictive – is that they may put the drug taker under pressures which lead to taking 'hard' drugs.

It is not only social dropouts and people with basic personality disorders who become drug addicts. Anyone whose job brings him into contact with dangerous drugs is at risk. A significant number of known addicts are doctors, nurses and midwives. Anyone working in the health services must be regarded as being at risk. The easiest way to control addiction might be to impose a total ban on all substances in the 'hard' drugs category but this is not desirable because it would mean the loss of several invaluable therapeutic agents. Instead, a system of controls is needed which distinguishes between medically useful and non-useful agents and permits, subject to limitations, their availability to the medical profession. Any such system of control must be able to classify dangerous drugs appropriately and while seeking to prevent the spread of addiction it must also protect existing addicts from exploitation and provide means whereby they may legally obtain supplies of drugs and, if possible, obtain treatment.

Poisons

Lethal poisons have been known to mankind since antiquity and classical history records their use for both suicidal and homicidal purposes. Before the mid-19th century deadly poisons such as arsenic and strychnine were more or less freely available to the public. They were used in a variety of ways, from poisoning rats and cleaning household objects to providing tonics for human use and medicine for specific diseases.

Arsenic as a poison

They were still being widely used for suicidal and homicidal purposes in the early and mid-Victorian era. A brief survey of famous murder cases of the time will soon show the popularity of poisoning and especially of using arsenic which produced symptoms not unlike those of a common condition, food poisoning. So great was the problem that Parliament in 1851 passed the Arsenic Act which for the first time imposed some statutory controls on the sale of this poison. Later the sales of other poisons were controlled, initially by the Pharmacy Act 1868 which introduced the first statutory poisons list.

Medical use of Poisons

The everyday use of poisons is less common today as modern and safer agents have been introduced but cyanide and arsenic in certain cases are still used to kill vermin, strychnine is still occasionally included in a 'tonic' and new poisons such as powerful disinfectants have been introduced. Although the medical use of poisons is small today their use as valuable cleansing and disinfecting agents continues – not least in the health services.

Poisons are 'Listed'

The hazards from poisons cannot be controlled unless they are listed and unless the list can be added to as new poisons are introduced. Such controls must limit the availability of the poisons to those who have a legitimate and reasonable use for them. Only in this way can the risks of homicidal, suicidal or accidental poisoning be minimised.

Modern Medicines – efficacy, quality and safety

Most modern medicines have made their appearance in the last 30 years and there are now specific and potent remedies for many diseases. However such modern drugs can produce a wide range of unwanted effects. Some of the effects may be no more than of nuisance value to the patient; others may be life-threatening.

Earlier in the history of therapeutics, when most medicines were palliative or ineffective they were also largely innocuous.

Today society demands that its medicines shall be both safe and effective, although in reality there can be no 'safe' drug which has any therapeutic effect. What must be achieved, therefore, is a balance between efficacy and safety, and obviously the more trivial the disease the higher the safety standard must be. Quality is also of vital importance. Modern medicines are complex chemical compounds usually formulated with inert substances into a form suitable for giving to the patients – tablets, capsules, injections and so on. The effectiveness of such treatment depends not only on the active ingredient but also the way in which it is formulated and the overall stability of that formulation. Two formulations of the same active drug may have different efficacy. It is therefore important to ensure that a medicinal product is of the right quality and capable of being reproduced in such a way that it has its planned effect every time it is used. Any set of controls on modern medicines must make a value judgment of the ratio of safety to efficacy of a potential new medicine in the light of the disease to be treated. It must prohibit the introduction of any medicine which fails to meet such ratios and must permit and encourage the speedy and efficient evaluation of potential new therapeutic agents. It must impose any restrictions necessary to ensure the safe use of medicines and a quality which will produce a uniform effect in patients.

Modern Systems of Legislation on Drugs, Poisons and Medicines

Any legislative system which imposes control on drugs, poisons and medicines must be comprehensive so that all foreseeable situations are dealt with. It must also be flexible so that it can adapt rapidly to changing circumstances. The law needs to be highly technical in parts and must have the support of relevant professional people. Finally, regulations should be introduced only after consultation with all interested parties; only in this way can a balance be struck between the necessary prohibitions and the necessary relaxations. A system of legislation known as delegated legislation has most of these characteristics and is the basis for the modern law in this area.

Delegated legislation

A large proportion of law today is statutory law – that is law made by Act of Parliament. In some cases an Act contains all of the newly introduced law and is self-contained. Such statutes are called constituent Acts. In other instances an Act merely gives someone (usually a Minister of the Crown) power to make within the broad scope of the Act regulations which have force of law. Such Statutes are called enabling Acts. The body of regulations they introduce is called delegated legislation and this is to be found in documents called Statutory Instruments. Statutes will usually be both constituent and enabling, introducing substantive law in some sections and enabling a body other than Parliament to introduce delegated legislation in other sections.

Enabling Acts are often used by Parliament for a variety of reasons. Shortage of Parliamentary time means it cannot introduce itself all the complex rules needed to regulate any modern society. Because Parliament is a lay body it is not qualified to introduce legislation of a highly technical nature.

The process of Parliamentary legislation does not involve detailed consultation with intertested parties. Indeed, a Parliamentary Bill (a draft Act) is a secret document until it is published for Parliamentary debate. Delegated legislation usually involves a consultative process. And finally, delegated legislation is flexible, allowing (insofar as the parent Act allows) new Statutory Instruments to be introduced as and when necessary.

Controls on delegated legislation

Under the British constitution only Parliament can make laws. Delegated legislation may seem to be an exception to this rule although, of course, the power to legislate is conferred by Parliament. Nonetheless, various checks and controls are imposed on delegated legislation to avoid possible administrative excesses.

Firstly, Parliament usually imposes limitations within the enabling Act on the extent to which a Minister may legislate, and often imposes a particular procedure that will bring the Statutory Instruments to the attention of Parliament either before or after they are introduced. Thus Section 10 of the Poisons Act 1972 provides that Statutory Instruments made under the Act may be annulled by resolution of either House of Parliament, and if the Minister wishes to change the Poisons List without the agreement of the Poisons Board he must lay the rules before Parliament together with his reason for wishing to proceed. Secondly there is a Scrutiny Committee of the House of Commons which reviews Statutory Instruments presented to Parliament.

On the other hand the courts may be used to challenge the validity of delegated legislation on the grounds that either it is outside the power conferred by the enabling Act or has been made without observing some important procedure laid down by the Act, such as a requirement for consultation. In such cases the courts may declare the delegated legislation to be 'ultra vires' – that is outside the power conferred by the Act and thus null and void.

The Modern Law on Drugs, Poisons and Medicines

The modern law on narcotic drugs, poisons and medicines is contained in three Acts of Parliament passed between 1968 and 1972. They are the Misuse of Drugs Act 1971, The Poisons Act 1972, and the Medicines Act 1968. All three statutes rely heavily on delegated legislation for their detailed regulations. For this reason, and because the introduction of some parts of one Act relate to the introduction of sections of others, their provisions have taken some years to introduce. Thus while the Medicines Act 1968 received the Royal Assent on 15th October 1968, the whole of the Act did not come into force until the end of 1978. The speed with which a large body of Statutory Instruments can be introduced is also related to the consultations with such interested parties as the British Medical Association and the Pharmaceutical Society. To keep abreast of the precise law in this area it is necessary to possess not only a copy of the relevant statutes but all of the Statutory Instruments, which should be obtained as they are published. HMSO publishes them, and its daily list of new publications is a useful way to spot their appearance.

Before dealing with the Acts in detail in later chapters it will be useful to review their broad scope here.

Misuse of Drugs Act 1971

This statute, which replaced the earlier Dangerous Drugs Acts, controls drugs of addiction and related abuse potential. The Act defines those drugs which it seeks to control and classifies them into categories based on the severity of their abuse potential. Broadly speaking the Act prohibits the import and export, production, supply and sale, and possession of such drugs. In so doing it creates a series of criminal offences for which it specifies penalties, which are themselves based on the category of drug involved in the offence.

To permit reasonable and necessary use of listed drugs by the medical and related professions (doctors, dentists, veterinarians and pharmacists, for example) the Act provides exceptions to the prohibitions. Thus either by regulations or the granting of a licence or both, a listed drug may be imported or manufactured, supplied to a doctor and possessed by a patient. However, in order to ensure that such relaxations are not abused, regulations exist to control such matters as the storage, inspection, labelling, and destruction of listed drugs and also to require that accurate records are kept. Penalties are provided for doctors who do not comply with these regulations.

There are provisions under the Act for known addicts to be registered and their drug supply to be maintained.

Finally the Act sets up an Advisory Council on the Misuse of Drugs which is made up mainly of members from the medical and allied professions. The council is required to keep under review the misuse of drugs in the UK and to advise the Ministers of any appropriate actions. It is also required to promote public knowledge of the hazards of drug abuse and to promote research into this field.

Poisons Act 1972

The Poisons Act 1972 replaces the Pharmacy and Poisons Act 1933, but unlike the earlier Act it extends only to non-medicinal products. Medicinal poisons (and non-poisons) are dealt with by the Medicines Act 1968.

The Poisons Act defines those substances it controls in the Poisons List which is divided into two parts. Part I poisons may be supplied only by a person conducting a retail pharmacy while Part II poisons may also be supplied by dealers on a local authority list. The Act provides for inspection of premises from which poisons are supplied.

To control the sale and supply of poisons and to ensure that where poison is supplied it is done so safely, a set of regulations known as the Poison Rules has been introduced. These rules control the mode of sale and supply, the storage, transport and labelling of poisons, the containers in which they may be put and their means of identification. The rules also provide for a system of record keeping.

The Act also provides for the establishment of a Poisons Board which has an advisory function with respect to additions to, and deletions from, the Poisons List and Rules.

Medicines Act 1968

The Medicines Act is the most complex and comprehensive of the modern Acts, and is associated with the greatest number of Statutory Instruments. It controls the manufacture, sale, supply and clinical trials of all medicinal products and applies to both human and veterinary medicines.

The Act controls these activities by a system of licences. Broadly speaking a licence is required to manufacture, supply, sell or promote medicinal products, to sell them wholesale or to do clinical studies with them. An administrative system exists to grant such licences provided certain requirements relating to safety, efficacy and quality have been satisfied.

A further means of control on medicinal products is the classification of them on the basis of whether they may be obtained only on prescription only, from a retail pharmacy or are generally available. The Act also controls the registration of retail pharmacies and provides that the British Pharmacopoeia (a dictionary of a wide variety of medicines) is a legal standard for the specification of those medicinal products.

Other legislation

While these three Acts cover nearly all the direct legislation on drugs, poisons and medicines, there is a large body of additional law indirectly concerned with this topic. For example, the Offences Against The Person Act 1861 prohibits the use of substances to procure an illegal abortion, and the Road Traffic Act 1972 deals with the offence of driving a motor vehicle while under the influence of drugs. Some of this additional legislation will also be dealt with in later chapters.

Chapter Two

MISUSE OF DRUGS ACT 1971

Controls on Dangerous Drugs

Introduction and Legal History

A broad outline of the problems associated with addictive drugs was given in Chapter 1, but before going into further detail certain terms will be defined and the categories of drugs outlined.

Definition of terms

The terms, addiction, dependence, habituation and abuse, when applied to drugs, are often used synonymously, and, while that is reasonable for the purposes of this book, one should be aware of certain implied differences in meaning.

Addiction is seen as the most severe form of the problem as for instance occurs with heroin.

Dependence is sometimes used to imply a less severe form of the condition as may be seen with the barbiturates. The form of the dependence may be psychological or physical. Psychological dependence is identified when, on withdrawal of the drug, emotional and subjective symptoms occur; physical dependence is recognised when physical symptoms of the withdrawal state occur as well.

Habituation covers the stage of the condition when drug-taking may be nothing more than a habit and therefore, with support, curable. The term, habituation, has been used to cover such things as tea and coffee drinking and cigarette smoking, although there have been many scientific discussions of whether such agents are addictive (albeit mildly so).

Drug abuse is a much wider term used to cover the whole range of problems. Literally interpreted it covers virtually any incorrect use of a drug; however this term is the one adopted by the legislature to describe the area of addiction and related phenomena.

Categories of Drugs

Many drugs and other substances are capable of producing true addiction and it has been suggested that any substance that alters how people feel will have an abuse potential. Certain types of drugs are of greater danger than others. Of greatest potential danger are the *narcotics,* a class of powerful pain killers derived from opium, either directly or by chemical manipulation. They include morphine, pethidine and heroin. Then there are the *psychotropic drugs,* drugs that have some effect on the emotional state. They include *stimulants* such as amphetamine, *depressants* such as the barbiturates and alcohol, and the *hallucinogens* such as lysergic acid diethylamide (LSD) and marihuana (cannabis, hashish, Indian hemp) which can produce mental hallucinations.

Although there is no doubt that both alcohol and the barbiturate drugs produce physical dependence, and nicotine in the form of tobacco smoke probably does so as well, tobacco, alcohol and barbiturates are not included in these drug abuse controls.

In 1972 the Advisory Council of the Misuse of Drugs considered the possibility of controls on barbiturates and concluded that a voluntary rather than legislative means of control should be adopted. Discussions with the medical profession led in 1975 to the Campaign on the Use and Restrictions of Barbiturates (CURB) which ran until 1977. The aim of the Campaign was to persuade the medical profession voluntarily to reduce the prescribing of barbiturates. Presently the Advisory Council is again considering legal methods of control.

Legal history of drug abuse controls

The law on drug abuse appeared late in legal history. In 1821 the famous 'opium eater', Thomas de Quincey, said, "What a man may lawfully seek in wine, surely he may find in opium," and this statement remained true for another 100 years. It was not until after the 1914-18 War that the sale of opium to the public was significantly controlled by law. The law has developed piecemeal, stimulated on the one hand by influences such as a series of International Agreements designed to control drug abuse and on the other by the changing face of the domestic 'drug scene'.

Perhaps the earliest control on drug abuse was the provision of the Poisons and Pharmacy Act 1908 which required a pharmacist to sell opium only to a person known to him. In 1912 an International Opium Convention was signed in the Hague but this was not introduced into UK law until after the 1914-18 War, when the Dangerous Drugs Act 1920 prohibited the import and export of opium for smoking and controlled the import and export of, and dealing with, narcotics. However, three years earlier, in 1917, it had been necessary to introduce wartime regulations prohibiting the supply of heroin, hemp, opium and morphine to troops without a doctor's prescription. This was due to the abuse of these agents then prevalent in the services.

The Dangerous Drugs Acts of 1923, 1925, 1932, 1950 and 1951 slowly extended the range of drugs brought under some legal control and culminated in the Dangerous Drugs Act 1965. Beside controlling all narcotics and cannabis, this gave effect to the Single Convention on Narcotic Drugs 1961 – an international agreement replacing earlier ones. However, these Acts were not comprehensive and several other statutes had to be introduced to control specific problems. Thus the Pharmacy and Poisons Act 1933 included narcotics and cannabis in the poisons rules (see page 33) and an amending Act of 1956 added amphetamines and barbiturates to the list. In 1964 it was necessary to enact the Drugs (Prevention of Misuse) Act to control the then prevalent misuse of amphetamines. However, as their availability was due to over prescribing by doctors, the problem was little improved, as the Act did nothing to control this. An amending Act of 1966 modified the 1964 Act to include LSD – a substance causing problems at that time. In 1967 a new step was taken in the Dangerous Drugs Act of that year which made the notification of heroin addicts compulsory, and controlled their drug supply.

By the end of the 1960s the law on drug misuse was spread over several Acts, and was inflexible and incomplete. The Misuse of Drugs Act 1971 was introduced to consolidate and strengthen the law into one single statute.

Misuse of Drugs Act 1971

The 1971 Act repeals the whole of the Drugs (Prevention of Misuse) Act 1964 and the Dangerous Drugs Acts 1965 and 1967. It applies to the whole of the United Kingdom.

Broadly speaking the Act does five things:

1) It lists the drugs to be controlled and classifies them for the purposes of the Act.
2) It prohibits virtually all activities with controlled drugs and thereby creates a series of criminal offences for which it specifies penalties and law enforcement procedures.

3) It authorises certain activities with controlled drugs for professional medical use (including dental and veterinary uses), which would otherwise be unlawful. However, these authorised activities are themselves subject to control.

4) It confers on the Secretary of State for the Home Department a variety of powers under the Act to prevent the misuse of drugs.

5) It creates the Advisory Council on the Misuse of Drugs.

The Act will now be considered under each of these broad heads.

The Controlled Drugs and their Classification

Classification for penalty purposes

Section 2 of the Act defines a controlled drug as any substance for the time being listed in Schedule 2 to the Act. Schedule 2 divides the listed drugs into three classes – A, B and C. The Act provides that Schedule 2 may be amended by Order in Council, after the draft order has been laid before Parliament and approved by a resolution of each House. An Order in Council is a form of delegated legislation in which, rather than the Minister making the regulation, it is nominally the Queen in Council who does so. This requirement is imposed by Parliament either where the subject matter of an order falls across the responsibility of several Ministers or where it is considered of sufficient importance to require the extra formality of such a process. The three classes of drugs relate to the penalties for their misuse and are based upon their perceived abuse potential.

Class A This contains the internationally controlled narcotics like morphine and opium, and the hallucinogens like LSD. Generally, maximum terms of imprisonment of seven years may be imposed for offences relating to possession of Class A drugs.

Class B This contains the amphetamine class, the codeine group of drugs and cannabis. However, any injectible form of a Class B drug is automatically in Class A. Maximum term of imprisonment for possession is five years.

Class C This contains the milder stimulants, and the maximum term of imprisonment for possession is two years.

Classification for the purpose of controls

While the above classification into different degrees of abuse potential is suitable for penalty determination, a classification that also reflects the therapeutic value of these drugs is required for setting limits on what medical use they may be put to. The Misuse of Drugs Regulations 1973 (SI 1973 No. 797), which lays down the conditions under which controlled drugs may be used medically, classifies them into four schedules for the purpose:

Schedule 1 This includes non-injectible preparations which contain such small quantities of controlled drugs (including morphine, cocaine, pholcodine and codeine) combined with other substances that they present a negligible abuse potential but are of therapeutic value. The recovery of the controlled drug from such preparations is most unlikely.

There are few controls on this group of preparations except that retailers must keep invoices for quantities they have obtained for two years, and producers and wholesalers must similarly retain invoices of quantities they have obtained and supplied.

Schedule 2 This includes the opiates, such as heroin, morphine and pethidine, and the major stimulants such as amphetamine. Activities with this category are stringently controlled. A licence is required for their import and export; they may be supplied by a pharmacist only on the authority of an appropriate practitioner, and there are requirements for labelling, safe custody, control of destruction and record-keeping.

Schedule 3 This includes the minor stimulants such as benzphetamine. Controls on this category are broadly similar to those under Schedule 2 but a little less stringent so that, for example, no entry is required in the register of controlled drugs and there is no control over their destruction.

Schedule 4 This includes substances of abuse potential which have virtually no accepted therapeutic use, but which may be used occasionally in research. They include the hallucinogens such as LSD and cannabis. Very stringent controls are imposed on them and they may be manufactured or used only under the authorisation of a licence issued by the Secretary of State.

Details of the controls imposed on each category of drug will be given in Chapter 3 (see page 20).

Restrictions on Controlled Drugs

The Act prohibits a variety of activities in respect of controlled drugs and thereby creates a series of criminal offences. The more important of these are:

Importation and exportation

Section 3 of the Act prohibits the importation and exportation of a controlled drug unless such activity has been authorised either by regulations made under Section 7 (see page 21) or by a licence issued by the Secretary of State. The actual offences of illegal import and export are created by the Customs and Excise Act 1952 and apply to Great Britain and Northern Ireland. The 1952 Act defines three offences – 'improper importation', contrary to Section 45 (1), 'improper exportation' contrary to Section 56 (2) and knowingly being involved in the evasion of 'importation and exportation prohibitions' contrary to Section 304. For Class A, B and C drugs, on summary conviction a penalty of three times the value of the goods or £400 fine, whichever is the greater, or 12 months imprisonment or both is possible. On conviction on indictment for Class A and B drugs imprisonment may be up to 14 years while with Class C up to five years.

Production and supply

Section 4 prohibits the production of controlled drugs and their supply to another, except under the authority of regulations made by the Secretary of State under the provisions of Section 7. The offences are 'illegally producing', or 'being concerned in the illegal production' of, a controlled drug, or 'supplying', 'offering to supply' or 'being concerned in the supplying' of a controlled drug to another. For Class A and B drugs on summary conviction a penalty of 12 months' imprisonment or £400 fine or both is available, while on indictment the penalty may be a term of 14 years or any fine or both. For Class C drugs on summary conviction the penalty may be six months imprisonment, £200 or both and on indictment five years imprisonment or any fine or both.

Possession

Section 5 prohibits the possession of a controlled drug unless it is authorised by regulations made under the provisions of Section 7. It is an offence to possess a controlled drug illegally, and to possess a controlled drug legally with the intent to supply to another contrary to Section 4 (above). There are two possible defences available to a charge of illegal possession – that, knowing or suspecting it to be a controlled drug, the accused took possession of it either to prevent another committing or continuing to commit a crime and that as soon as reasonably possible took all reasonable steps to destroy the drug or deliver it to a person lawfully entitled to take custody of it or to deliver it to such a person and as soon as possible took all reasonable steps to do so (S 5(4)(b)). Thus any health service staff who may take charge of what they believe is a controlled drug should deliver it to a doctor or pharmacist or to the police as soon as possible or they may not be able to rely on this defence.

Illegal possession of Class A drugs carries a 12 month term or a £400 fine or both on summary conviction, and seven years' imprisonment or any fine or both on indictment. With Class B drugs the fines are the same but the maximum term of imprisonment on summary conviction is six months, and five years on indictment. For Class C drugs on summary conviction it is six months' imprisonment or £200 fine or both, and two years' imprisonment or any fine or both on indictment. Possession with intent to supply carries higher penalties – for example, 14 years on indictment for Class A and B drugs.

Cannabis

Section 6 of the Act prohibits the cultivation of any plant of the genus Cannabis unless authorised by regulations or a licence issued by the Secretary of State. Illegal cultivation on summary conviction may be punished with 12 months' imprisonment or £400 fine or both, and, on indictment, with 14 years or any fine or both.

Miscellaneous offences

In order to strengthen the prohibitions in Sections 3, 4, 5 & 6 of the Act certain other offences are defined. Thus Section 9 prohibits the smoking of opium, the possession of pipes or utensils used in connection with opium smoking, and the frequenting of any place for this purpose. Section 8 makes it an offence for the occupier of, or person concerned in the management of, premises knowingly to permit certain activities to take place there. These activities are illegal production, or an attempt thereat, of a controlled drug; illegal supply, attempt to supply or offering to supply a controlled drug; preparing opium for smoking, or the smoking of cannabis, cannabis resin or opium.

For class A and B drugs on summary conviction there may be 12 months' imprisonment or a £400 fine or both while on indictment the penalty may be up to 14 years' imprisonment or any fine or both. For class C drugs the figures are six months or £200 fine or both on summary conviction and 5 years or any fine or both on indictment.

People involved in hospital management are certainly 'concerned with the management of premises' for the purpose of these offences. A hospital resident, say a doctor or nurse living in hospital accommodation, is likely to be an 'occupier' for the purpose of the offences. In *R v Tao 1976* it was held that an undergraduate occupying a room at a college hostel in which cannabis was smoked was an occupier as he had exclusive possession of the room.

Section 19 makes it an offence to *attempt* to commit any offence under the Act or to incite or attempt to incite any offence under the Act. Section 21 provides that where the offence is committed by a corporation, if the offence was with the consent or connivance of, or due to the neglect of, a director, manager, secretary or similar official that person shall also be guilty of that offence.

Sections 23 and 24 provide powers of search and arrest for the police and makes it an offence to obstruct police who are investigating a suspected offence under the Act. Section 27 provides that *anything* related to the offence may be forfeit on order of the Court for destruction, or to be dealt with in other appropriate manner.

Authorised Dealings with Controlled Drugs

The prohibitions and related offences described above are clearly necessary to reduce and prevent the misuse of controlled drugs. However, they also place unacceptable restrictions on certain categories of valuable agents. To solve this conflict of interests the Act permits the Secretary of State to authorise people in the medical and allied professions to do things in respect of controlled drugs that would otherwise be unlawful. The following section describes in general terms these relaxations, and chapter 3 gives a detailed account of them.

Regulations to permit the professional use of controlled drugs

Section 7 permits the Secretary of State to make regulations that authorise certain individuals to import, export, produce, supply or possess certain controlled drugs, or to cultivate cannabis. These regulations may authorise such activities directly to a class of people, or by licence to an individual or group, and Section 30 provides that such licences may be subject to such terms and conditions as the Secretary of State thinks appropriate (including the payment of a fee). Section 31 provides that in making regulations the Secretary of State may distinguish between different controlled drugs, or different classes of person; may make the opinion, consent or approval of a third party material for the provision of a regulation, and may make transitional arrangements. Sections 7 and 31 also provide that the Secretary of State must consult with the Advisory Council (see page 19) before making regulations and that these regulations may be annulled by resolution of either House of Parliament.

Section 7 directs the Secretary of State to make regulations that will make it not unlawful for a doctor, dentist or veterinarian (i.e. a 'practitioner'), acting in their capacity as such, to supply a controlled drug, and for a pharmacist or someone lawfully conducting a retail pharmacy business to manufacture, compound or supply controlled drugs. Regulations have also been made making it not unlawful for a doctor, dentist, veterinarian or pharmacist, acting in his capacity as such, to have a controlled drug in their possession. Notwithstanding these directions to the Secretary of State, Section 7(4)(a) and (b) permits him to make the production, supply and possession of certain drugs wholly unlawful, or unlawful except for research purposes if it is in the public interest to do so.

Similarly he may make it unlawful for practitioners and pharmacists to have any dealings with certain drugs unless under the specific authority of a licence. In this way the Act generally, and Section 7(4)(b) in particular, limits the right of a practitioner to prescribe whatever drug he chooses.

Regulations to prevent the misuse of controlled drugs

Having made provisions in Section 7 for practitioners to have access to certain controlled drugs for therapeutic purposes the Act proceeds to impose a variety of controls to avoid these provisions being a source of misuse.

Section 10 directs the Secretary of State to make regulations covering the following; safe custody of controlled drugs, documentation of transactions involving controlled drugs, keeping of records and furnishing of information, inspection of precautions and records, packing and labelling of controlled drugs, issue of prescriptions for controlled drugs, notification of drug addicts, and prohibition on doctors prescribing for addicts except under the provisions of a licence issued by the Secretary of State. This latter item is another example of a doctor's freedom to prescribe being limited.

Offences related to the professional use of controlled drugs

Section 12 deals with the practitioner or pharmacist who has been convicted under the Act, the Dangerous Drugs Act 1965 or those sections of the Customs and Excise Act 1952 that prohibit the import and export of controlled drugs. In such circumstances the Secretary of State may prohibit the practitioner from possessing, prescribing, administering, manufacturing, compounding or supplying controlled drugs. Section 13(2) provides that the Secretary of State may issue such a prohibition where he is of the opinion that a practitioner is prescribing, administering, supplying or authorising the administration or supply of any controlled drugs in an irresponsible way.

Failure to comply with a direction issued by the Secretary of State under either Section 12 or Section 13 is an offence which, for class A and B drugs, on summary conviction may carry a term of imprisonment of 12 months or £400 fine or both, and on indictment 14 years, any fine or both. For class C drugs, on summary conviction the penalty is six months' imprisonment or £200 or both while on indictment five years or any fine or both.

Investigations and tribunals

Although the Secretary of State is free to make a direction under Section 13(1) or (2) without reference to any other body, Section 14 provides that he may refer the case to a special tribunal which consists of five people. One of these is a lawyer appointed by the Lord Chancellor and is chairman. The other four are appointed by the Secretary of State from members of the practitioner's profession. While this procedure is not mandatory, it is expected that the Secretary of State will normally follow it. If the tribunal finds that there has been no contravention of regulations or irresponsible prescribing, it advises the Secretary of State accordingly and he must inform the practitioner. If the tribunal finds the practitioner at fault the Secretary of State must serve notice of such findings on the practitioner who has 28 days to make representations to him. If representations are made the Secretary of State must refer the case to an advisory body made up of three people one of whom is a Queen's Counsel appointed by the Lord Chancellor to be chairman. The other two are members of the practitioner's profession – one from a Government Department and one from the practitioner's professional body. The advisory body must advise the Secretary of State in the exercise of his powers.

Where the Secretary of State believes that there has been irresponsible prescribing and wishes to issue a prohibition under Section 13(2) without delay he may do so under provisions of Section 15. He may issue a temporary direction that is effective for six weeks from its service on the practitioner. In such a case the Secretary of State *must* refer the case to a professional panel and give the practitioner a chance of appearing and being heard. The professional panel is made up of three members – a chairman and two others all appointed from the practitioner's profession. If the panel advises that there has not been irresponsible prescribing then the temporary direction is cancelled. If the panel advises that the case is established then the direction is made permanent.

Powers of Investigation of the Secretary of State

The powers vested in the Secretary of State to make regulations, issue licences and to limit the right of individual practitioners to prescribe have already been described. Section 17 gives the Secretary of State a variety of powers to obtain information from practitioners and pharmacists relating to the misuse of drugs. If there appears to be a social problem in a particular part of Great Britain related to the misuse of drugs the Secretary of State may require any doctor or pharmacist in that area to furnish him with details of drug usage there. Failure to comply with such a request for information is an offence. It is also an offence to supply false information. Failure to comply carries a penalty of £100 fine on summary conviction. For giving false information there may be a term of imprisonment of six months or £400 fine or both on summary conviction, and on indictment two years or any fine or both.

The Advisory Council on the Misuse of Drugs

An Advisory Council is established under Section 1 of the Act. There must be at least 20 members and their appointment is made by the Home Secretary after consultations with the various professional bodies. There must be at least one person with wide and recent experience of medicine, dentistry, veterinary medicine, pharmacy, the pharmaceutical industry and chemistry. There must also be members with wide and recent experience of social problems associated with the misuse of drugs. These would include, for example, psychiatrists, social workers and educationalists.

Functions of the Advisory Council

Review The Council is required to keep under review the total situation with respect to drug misuse in the United Kingdom. It must give appropriate advice to the 'Ministers' when the Council think it expedient to do so, or when consulted. Such advice may contain a recommendation to change the law. The 'Ministers' are the Secretary of State for the Home Department, the Secretaries of State concerned with health in England, Wales and Scotland, the Secretaries of State concerned with education in England, Wales and Scotland, the Minister for Home Affairs for Northern Ireland, the Minister of Health and Social Services for Northern Ireland and the Minister of Education for Northern Ireland.

Advisory The Council must advise the 'Ministers' on any matter related to drug abuse that is referred to it.

Education and research The Council must pay particular attention in the review of potential drug abuse to the education of the public and especially young people concerning the dangers of drugs. It must also promote research into all aspects of the problem. The Council is required to address itself to the problem of promoting co-operation between the professions and the various community services, and also to ensuring that proper advice, treatment and rehabilitation are available to addicts.

Regulations The Secretary of State must consult with the Council before altering the list of controlled drugs (Section 2(2)), limiting the availability of controlled drugs to research purposes only (Section 7(4)), or making any regulation under the Act.

Chapter Three

MISUSE OF DRUGS ACT 1971

Regulations: Practical Aspects

In chapter 2 the prohibitions on import, export, production, possession and supply of controlled drugs set out in Sections 3-6 of the 1971 Act were described. The direction in s7 to the Secretary of State for the Home Department to make such regulations as are necessary to permit the medical and related use of such drugs was also described. Section 10 requires regulations to be made to control the activities with controlled drugs authorised by s7. Section 22 empowers the Secretary of State to make any such regulations applicable to servants or agents of the Crown.

In this chapter we will consider the practical implications of those regulations made so far. These regulations fall under four more or less well defined heads:

> Regulations making lawful what would otherwise be unlawful ('Section 7 regulations');
>
> regulations concerning the destruction of controlled drugs;
>
> regulations concerning their safe custody, and
>
> regulations concerning the notification of drug addicts and their supplies.

The regulations will be dealt with under these four headings.

It was mentioned in chapter 2 that the Misuse of Drugs Regulations 1973 (as amended) SI 1973 No 797 categorises controlled drugs into four groups which are relevant to the application of these regulations. They are as follows:

Schedule 1 Controlled drugs compounded with other substances in such small quantities that they are unlikely to be of danger.

Schedule 2 The opiates and major stimulants.

Schedule 3 The minor stimulants.

Schedule 4 Hallucinogenic agents (for example, LSD) and cannabis which have no established therapeutic value.

Section 7 Regulations – Authorisation of Activities Otherwise Unlawful

The following regulations are contained in the Misuse of Drugs Regulations 1973 pt II as amended (SI 1973 No 797).

Production, supply and possession for medical purposes

a) Schedule 1 drugs
Sections 3(1) and 5(1) of the Act prohibit the import, export and possession of controlled drugs but do not apply to Schedule 1 drugs.

b) Licences to produce etc. a controlled drug
A person authorised by the Secretary of State by licence to do so may produce, supply, offer for sale or have in his possession a controlled drug without committing an offence under the Act. This is assuming the provisions and conditions of the licence are complied with. In practice this applies mainly to manufacturers. A hospital would not normally need a licence as regulations permit doctors and pharmacists to manufacture and compound Schedule 1, 2 and 3 drugs (see below).

c) General authority to possess
General authority to have in his or her possession a controlled drug is given to;

(i) a police constable acting in the course of his duty,
(ii) a carrier acting as such,
(iii) a post office employee in the course of his duty,
(iv) a customs and excise officer acting in his capacity as such,
(v) someone working in a forensic laboratory where a drug has been sent for analysis and acting in the course of his duty,
(vi) someone engaged in conveying the drug to someone authorised to possess it.

d) Administration of controlled drugs (reg. 7)
Any person irrespective of qualification may administer a Schedule 1 drug to any other person provided no other offence is committed (see chapter 9). A doctor or dentist or someone acting under the direction of a doctor or dentist may administer any drug in schedule 2 or 3 to any patient. This assumes that the

Secretary of State has not withdrawn this authority from the practitioner under the powers in s13 or s15 of the Act (see page 17) and the patient is not a registered addict when a licence may be required to prescribe (see page 31). Schedule 4 substances may not be administered by anyone who does not possess a special licence to do so issued by the Secretary of State. Such licences are issued only for research and scientific purposes.

e) Production and supply of Schedule 1, 2 and 3 drugs (reg. 8 & 9)

A practitioner or pharmacist acting in his capacity as such may *manufacture or compound* any drug in Schedule 1, 2 or 3. Similarly a person lawfully conducting a retail pharmacy business (see page 72) and acting in that capacity may also do so at the pharmacy where he carries on business.

Provided he or she is acting in his or her capacity as such, any one of the following may supply or offer to supply a Schedule 1, 2 or 3 drug to any person who may lawfully possess it:

(i) A practitioner, pharmacist or person conducting a retail pharmacy business.

(ii) The matron or acting matron of a hospital or nursing home wholly or mainly maintained by public funds or a charity. At any other type of hospital or home only a Schedule 3 drug is covered.

(iii) A sister or acting sister in charge of a ward, theatre or other department in a hospital or nursing home, where the drug is supplied to him or her by a person responsible for dispensing and supply of medicines in that hospital.

(iv) Someone in charge of a laboratory attached to a hospital, university or other institution approved by the Secretary of State whose recognised activities are scientific, educational or research. Schedule 1, 2 and 3 drugs are covered in the case of a recognised institution whereas only Schedule 3 drugs are covered for institutions not attached to a University or hospital.

(v) A public analyst appointed under the Food and Drugs Act 1955 or the Food and Drugs (Scotland) Act 1956.

(vi) A sampling officer under the Acts in (v) above or under the Medicines Act 1968.

(vii) Someone engaged in a scheme to test the quality of drugs supplied to the National Health Service under the National Health Service Acts 1949-73 or the equivalent Act in Scotland.

However, a matron or acting matron may supply or offer to supply a drug only where there is no pharmacist responsible for dispensing in that hospital or nursing home. Also, a sister or acting sister in charge of a ward etc. may supply a drug only for administration to a patient in that ward etc. and under the direction of a doctor or dentist.

In addition to these provisions which cover the health service the regulations also permit the master or owner of a ship which does not carry a doctor, and the manager of an offshore installation, to supply controlled drugs to a crew man.

f) Possession of controlled drugs (reg. 10)
There is no restriction on a Schedule 1 drug.

Those categories listed under (i) to (vii) above may possess Schedule 2 and 3 drugs, with the same distinction between Schedule 2 and 3 as is made in (ii) and (iv) above. The owner or master of a ship not carrying a doctor, the master of a foreign ship in a British port or the manager of an offshore installation may possess Schedule 2 and 3 drugs insofar as it is necessary to fulfil their legal duties.

Any person may have in his or her possession a Schedule 2 or 3 drug for administration for medical, dental or veterinary use under the directions of a practitioner, provided it was not obtained under false pretences.

g) Pethidine and midwives (reg. 11)
A midwife certified under the Midwives Act 1951 or the Midwives (Scotland) Act 1951 who has notified the area health authority of her intention to practise may possess and administer pethidine insofar as is necessary for the practice of midwifery, and may surrender to her appropriate medical officer any stocks no longer required by her. A midwife may lawfully possess only pethidine she has obtained on a midwife's supply order signed by the area medical officer. A midwife's supply order must specify in writing the name and occupation of the midwife, the purpose for which the drug is required and the total quantity required.

h) Cannabis (reg. 12 & 13)
The Secretary of State may issue a licence to authorise the cultivation of plants of the genus Cannabis. He may also approve premises for the smoking of cannabis or cannabis resin for research purposes.

Requirements Concerning Documentation

a) Supplies of Schedule 2 and 3 drugs other than on prescription

(i) Supplies to practitioners (reg. 14)
Where controlled drugs are supplied other than on prescription to a practitioner, a matron or acting matron of a hospital or nursing home, someone in charge of a recognised scientific, educational or research

WARD RECORD BOOK
CONTROLLED DRUGS

NAME, FORM OF PREPARATION AND STRENGTH ....

AMOUNT(S) OBTAINED			AMOUNTS ADMINISTERED							
Amount	Date Received	Serial No. of Requis-ition	Date	Time	Patient's Name	Amount Given	Given by (Signature)	Witnessed by (Signature)	STOCK BALANCE

WARD REQUISITION
ORDER FOR CONTROLLED DRUGS

Serial No. ....

.... *Hospital*

Ward or Department ....

Name of Preparation	Strength	Quantity

(Each preparation to be ordered on a separate page)

Ordered by .... *Date* ....
(Signature of Sister or Acting Sister)

Supplied by.. *Date* ....
(Pharmacist's Signature)

Accepted for delivery .... *Date* ....
(Signature of Messenger)

laboratory or the owner or master of a ship without a doctor, a master of a foreign ship in a British port or the manager of an offshore installation, the supplier must obtain a requisition in writing. The requisition must be signed by the recipient giving his name, address and profession. It must specify the use to which the drug is to be put and the total quantity to be supplied. Before supplying the material the supplier must be reasonably satisfied that the signature and declared profession are genuine.

Where a practitioner is unable to furnish the supplier with a requisition because the drug is required urgently by reason of some emergency, the supplier may let the recipient have the material if he is satisfied that this is a bona fide emergency. In such a case the practitioner must undertake to provide a proper requisition within 24 hours.

A requisition from the matron etc. of a hospital etc. must be signed by a doctor or dentist working there.

(ii) Third parties collecting supplies

Where the potential recipient of controlled drugs under a requisition sends someone on his behalf to collect the material from the supplier, the supplier shall not deliver the drug to that person unless he produces an authority to receive the material on the recipient's behalf signed by the recipient. The supplier may hand over the material only if he is satisfied that the document is genuine.

(iii) Supplies from a hospital dispensary to a ward

A requisition is required where the person responsible in a hospital or nursing home for the dispensing and supply of medicines supplies a controlled drug to a sister or acting sister in charge of a ward, theatre or other department. The requisition must be in writing signed by the recipient and specifying the total quantity of drug to be supplied. The requisition must be marked by the supplier as complied with (to stop it being used twice) and retained in the dispensary. The recipient must also keep a copy. A typical ward requisition form is shown on the facing page.

b) Supplies on Prescription

(i) Correct form of prescription (reg. 15)

A prescription for a controlled drug in Schedule 2 or 3 must be indelible, and signed and dated by the person issuing it. The issuer must, also in his own handwriting, specify the name and address of the person for whose treatment it is issued, and the dose to be taken, the strength of the preparation and the total quantity to be supplied. Numerical data (for example, the dose) must be both in figures and words to prevent alteration. The prescription must state the address of the person issuing it if it is not a NHS prescription (for example, a veterinary one). If it is issued by a dentist it must be marked "for dental treatment only", and if issued by a veterinarian "for animal treatment only". If the prescription envisages the material to be dispensed in instalments it must state the amount of each instalment and their intervals.

If the prescription is for the treatment of a patient in hospital or a nursing home it is not necessary to include the name and address of the person treated if the prescription is written on the patient's card or case notes.

These requirements do not apply to prescriptions issued under a NHS testing scheme for sampling the quality of drugs supplied to the Service.

(ii) Supply on prescription (reg. 16)

Before a Schedule 2 or 3 drug may be supplied on prescription the supplier must ensure the form of the prescription is correct (as above), that the address of the issuer is in the UK and that he is familiar with the signature. He should have no reason to suspect the signature is not genuine or if necessary take steps to ensure it is so. The prescription must not be issued before the date on it, and not later than 13 weeks after. When the drug is dispensed the prescription must be marked with the date of dispensing, and if it is not a NHS prescription it must be retained on the premises. In the case of a prescription directing instalments of drugs to be dispensed the dispenser must follow that direction. In such a case the first instalment must be within 13 weeks and each time an instalment is supplied it must be marked on the prescription.

These requirements do not apply to a NHS quality testing scheme.

c) The marking of bottles etc. (reg. 18)

Where a controlled drug in Schedule 2 or 3 is supplied it must be in a bottle, package or other container that is clearly marked either with the amount of drug therein, or, if it is compounded into tablets, capsules etc., the number of dose units and the amount of drug in each. However, this requirement does not apply to supply on a practitioners prescription.

d) Drug registers (reg. 19 & 20)

Anyone authorised to supply Schedule 2 or 4 drugs must in respect of those drugs keep a register in which are entered in chronological order details of the quantity of drugs both obtained and supplied. Separate registers or a separate part of the register must be kept for each class of drug. Such a register need not be kept by the sister or acting sister of a ward or other department, although this is not to say that a ward register is a bad idea.

The following rules must be observed in maintaining the register:

(i) Each page should indicate at its head which class of drugs it refers to.

(ii) Entries must be made on the day of the transaction or, where that is impossible, at the very latest on the next day.

(iii) There must be no cancellations, alterations, or obliterations. Corrections must be made by way of a dated footnote or marginal note.

(iv) All entries must be indelible.

(v) The register must not be used for any other purpose.

The person keeping the register must show it to any person authorised in writing by the Secretary of State, and give details of any registered transaction. He must also show his stocks to the authorised person if required to do so.

A register must be kept at each of the premises where the business or occupation is carried on in respect of transactions at those premises. The prescribed form of register is shown on the next page.

e) The midwife's register (reg. 21)

A midwife authorised to have pethidine in her possession (see page 23) must keep a book in which she enters the date of acquisition of all supplies together with the name and address of the supplier and the amount and form obtained. When she gives pethidine to a patient she must as soon as practicable enter the name and address of the patient, the amount given and the form used. The form of register shown on the next page is also suitable for midwives' use.

f) Preservation of records

All registers and midwives' books must be kept for a period of two years from the last entry. Similarly every requisition, order or prescription (other than a NHS prescription) on which controlled drugs are supplied must be kept for a period of two years from the date when the last delivery was made.

FORM OF REGISTER

PART I

Entries to be made in case of obtaining

Date on which supply received	NAME	ADDRESS	Amount obtained	Form in which obtained
	Of person or firm from whom obtained			

PART II

Entries to be made in case of supply

Date on which the transaction was effected	NAME	ADDRESS	Particulars as to licence or authority of person or firm supplied to be in possession	Amount supplied	Form in which supplied
	Of person or firm supplied				

Requirements Concerning Destruction

One possible source of illegal controlled drugs could be material that has falsely been claimed to have been destroyed – because, for instance, it had passed the manufacturer's expiry date. Regulation 24 seeks to control this abuse. No-one who is required to keep records with respect to Schedule 2 or 4 drugs may destroy or cause them to be destroyed except in the presence of, and under the direction of, a person authorised by the Secretary of State.

Persons authorised by the Secretary of State include police constables, Pharmaceutical Society Inspectors and Home Office Drugs Branch Inspectors (HO circular 78/1973).

The person keeping the records must enter the date and quantity destroyed, and this must be signed by the authorised person. The authorised person may take a sample of the drug for analysis to ensure it was indeed a controlled drug.

Safe Custody of Controlled Drugs

It is clearly important that controlled drugs be stored securely and the Misuse of Drugs (Safe Custody) Regulations 1973 (SI 1973 No 798), as amended, provides rules for their safe custody.

a) Special safe custody requirements (reg. 3)

Special safe custody requirements apply to controlled drugs stored on the following premises:

(i) A retail dealer (ie a retail pharmacy business or a pharmacist supplying drugs to the public at a health centre within the meaning of the Medicines Act 1968).

(ii) A nursing home as defined by part VI of the Public Health Act 1936 or the Nursing Homes Registration (Scotland) Act 1938.

(iii) Any residential establishment under s59 of the Social Work (Scotland) Act 1968.

(iv) Any nursing home as defined by part III of the Mental Health Act 1959.

(v) Any private hospital under the Mental Health (Scotland) Act 1960.

The occupier and every person concerned in the management of these premises must ensure that all controlled drugs are kept in a locked safe, cabinet or room constructed and maintained so as to prevent unauthorised access. Schedule 2 to the regulations defines in detail the construction of suitable safes, cabinets and rooms.

There are certain exceptions to these special requirements for safe custody as follows:

(i) In the case of a retail dealer where the drugs are for the time being under the direct personal supervision of the pharmacist, or in the case of other premises under the direct personal supervision of the person in charge of the drugs or a member of the staff appointed for the purpose.

(ii) In the case of a retail dealer a certificate may be obtained from the Chief Officer of police in the area exempting him from the scheduled constructional requirements. To do so the Chief Officer must inspect the premises and certify that the storage facilities are of an "adequate degree of security".

(iii) Drugs listed in Schedule 1 to the Misuse of Drugs Regulations 1973 and the extra ones listed in Schedule 1 to the Misuse of Drugs (Safe Custody) Regulations 1973.

b) General requirements (reg. 5)

Where controlled drugs are stored other than on the premises listed above and not in a locked safe, cabinet or room then the person having possession of them must ensure that as far as possible they are kept in a locked receptacle which can be opened only by him or someone authorised by him.

This requirement does not apply to:

(i) Drugs in Schedule 1 of the Misuse of Drugs Regulations 1973 and the extra drugs listed in Schedule 1 to the Misuse of Drugs (Safe Custody) Regulations 1973.

(ii) Persons to whom the drug is supplied on prescription.

(iii) A carrier or someone engaged in the business of the Post Office.

Notification of and Supply to Addicts

The Misuse of Drugs (Notification of and Supply to Addicts) Regulations 1973 (SI 1973 No 799) introduces a system whereby doctors are under a duty to notify people who are, or are suspected of being, addicted to certain controlled drugs. These drugs are cocaine dextromoramide, heroin (Diamorphine), dipipanone, hydrocodone, hydromorphone, levorphanol, methadone, morphine, opium, oxycodone, pethidine, phenazocine or piritramide.

a) Notification

Where a doctor considers, or has reasonable grounds to suspect, that someone is addicted to one of the drugs listed above he must inform the Chief Medical Officer of the Home Office within seven days in writing and specify the person's name, address, sex, date of birth, NHS number, date of attendance and name of drug involved.

The regulations provide that a person is to be regarded as addicted to a drug "if, and only if, he has as a result of repeated administration become so dependent upon that drug that he has an overpowering desire for the administration of it to be continued."

Notification is not necessary:

(i) where continued administration of the drug is to treat an organic disease or injury;

(ii) where notification has been made in the last 12 months by that doctor, another in the same practice or if the attendance is at a hospital by another doctor at that hospital.

b) Restrictions on prescribing for addicts

Where a doctor considers, or has reasonable cause to suspect, a person is addicted to any of the drugs listed above he must *not* administer, supply or prescribe either cocaine or heroin to that person.

This restriction does not apply:

(i) if the drug is used to treat organic disease or injury,

(ii) is given in accordance with a licence issued by the Secretary of State, or

(iii) if authorised by another doctor holding an appropriate licence.

In practice drug addicts are treated at addiction centres, usually in the charge of consultant psychiatrists who will be licensed by the Home Office to supply addicts.

Summary

The table below gives a broad summary of the controls on scheduled drugs imposed by the Misuse of Drugs Regulations 1973. Details will be found earlier in the chapter.

SUMMARY OF MISUSE OF DRUGS REGULATIONS 1973

ACTIVITY REGULATED	SCHEDULE 1	SCHEDULE 2	SCHEDULE 3	SCHEDULE 4
Import and export	no controls	by licence only		
Production	by pharmacists, retail pharmacy business, practitioner or by licence.			by licence only
Supply	by practitioner, pharmacist, retail pharmacy business, matron if no pharmacist, sister on a ward and by licence			by licence only
Possession	no control	licence holder, policeman, carrier, PO employee, customs and excise officer, forensic laboratory.		
		practitioner, pharmacist, retail pharmacy business, matron if no pharmacist and ward sister.		
Prescription	no	yes		by licence only
Requisitions	no	yes		
Administration	no control	by doctor, dentist or someone acting under their instructions		by licence only
Drug register	no	yes	no	yes
Labelling	no	yes		
Safe custody	no	yes		
Destruction	no	yes	no	yes

Chapter Four

THE POISONS ACT 1972

Controls on Poisons

Introduction and History

Until the mid-nineteenth century there were no legal controls on the sale of poisons to the public. From that time to the present day the modern law on poisons has built up, and its development has gone hand in hand with the development of pharmacy as a profession. Indeed, most of the statutes involving poisons have included provisions regulating the practice of pharmacy. With the advent of modern medicines from the 1940s, the poisons law together with the Therapeutic Substances Acts were the only controls on these new substances (assuming they were not caught by the dangerous drugs legislation). Today the law on poisons concerns only non-medicinal poisons; medicinal poisons are included in the provisions of the Medicines Act 1968. This chapter and the next therefore deal only with non-medicinal poisons.

The earliest poisons control was contained in the Arsenic Act 1851, but it was not until 1868 that the Pharmacy Act introduced a poisons list and controlled the sales of items listed on it. The first poisons list included 15 substances and the Act empowered the Pharmaceutical Society to add to the list as they deemed fit. Listed poisons could only be sold either by a 'pharmaceutical chemist' or a 'chemist and druggist'. A pharmaceutical chemist was someone who had passed the pharmacy examinations set by the Pharmaceutical Society under the provisions of the Pharmacy Act 1832. This qualification was known as the 'major exam' to distinguish it from the examination set up by the 1868 Act for the title of chemist and druggist and called the 'minor exam'. This distinction between types of pharmacist continued until 1953. The 1869 Pharmacy Act also regulated the labelling of poisons and the manner in which they could be sold.

Breaches of the Act led to fixed penalties that were recoverable in the civil courts.

The Poisons and Pharmacy Act 1908 extended the poisons list and made provision that agricultural and horticultural poisons could be sold by licensed dealers as well as pharmacists. The Act also empowered a corporate body to carry on a pharmacy business – a step necessary to reverse the decision in *Pharmaceutical Society v London and Provincial Supply Association Ltd 1880* where it was held that a company was not a 'Person' for the purposes of the 1868 Act.

The Pharmacy and Poisons Act 1933 extended the poisons list considerably and classified it into many subsections each with its own set of controls. Listed poisons could be sold only by a pharmacy or someone on a special local authority list. A Poisons Board was established to have an advisory function in the application of the Act. The Pharmaceutical Society was to enforce the Act and breaches were to be proceeded against in courts of summary jurisdiction (for example, magistrates courts) rather than in the civil courts as previously. The Act also dealt with the regulation of the profession of pharmacy, requiring all pharmacists to be members of the Pharmaceutical Society and establishing a disciplinary body.

As mentioned earlier, the 1933 Act was for over 40 years the only control on some new medicinal products, covering as it did both medicinal and non-medicinal poisons. However, the Medicines Act 1968 was enacted among other things to control the sale of all types of medicinal products. These controls (part III of the Medicines Act) were introduced in 1978 and from the same date the provisions of the Poisons Act 1972 came into force.

The Poisons Act 1972

The Poisons Act 1972 deals only with non-medicinal poisons. These are defined by s11 as substances included in the Poisons List (see page 36) which are not medicinal products as defined by s130 of the Medicines Act 1968 (page 52) nor have been brought under the control of that Act by an order under s104 or s105. These sections cover articles and substances which are not strictly medicinal products as defined but are used either for a medicinal purpose or as an ingredient in a medicinal product. The 1972 Act does not extend to Northern Ireland.

Therefore, however toxic a substance may be it is not a poison for the purpose of this Act if it is not on the Poisons List. Conversely, if a substance is on the list any preparation containing that substance will also be considered a poison unless a specific exemption is given, however small the quantity is. This has not always been the case, however. Although in *Pharmaceutical Society of Great Britain v Piper & Co. 1893* it was held that chlorodyne, a preparation containing morphine, a poison listed by the Pharmacy Act 1868, was itself a poison, in the same year it was held in *Pharmaceutical Society of Great Britain v Delve 1893* that the preparation Licoricine was not a poison. This was because although it contained morphine it was present in infinitesimal quantities. Today, however, any substance containing a listed poison in any quantity is itself a poison unless exempted by the Poison Rules or List.

Broadly speaking the Act deals with four related aspects of poisons controls – the establishment of a Poisons Board, the listing of controlled poisons, controls on the sale of listed poisons, and a system of inspection to enforce the provisions of the Act. The Act will be dealt with in the rest of this chapter under these four heads, and the detailed requirements of the Poisons Rules will be discussed in the next chapter.

The Poisons Board

Section 1 of the Poisons Act confirms the existence of an advisory committee called the Poisons Board (set up under the 1933 Act) and provides that it may establish its own constitution subject to approval by the Secretary of State for the Home Department. The Board must advise the Secretary of State on matters concerning poisons and s10 provides that if the Secretary of State intends to vary the Poisons List or make rules under the Act and the Poisons Board do not concur with such action he must lay the proposals before both Houses of Parliament together with a statement of why he wishes to proceed. Such an order may be annulled by resolution of either House of Parliament whether or not the order has the support of the Board.

The constitution of the Board is outlined in Schedule 1 to the Act. It consists of 16 members, and the Secretary of State may from time to time appoint three extra members. Five members are appointed by – the Secretary of State for the Home Department (1), the Secretary of State for Scotland (1), the Secretary of State for Social Services (2) and the Minister of Agriculture, Fisheries and Food (1). The Government Chemist is a member. Five are appointed by the Council of the Pharmaceutical Society, and one each by the Royal College of Physicians of London, the equivalent College in Edinburgh, the General Medical Council, the Council of the Royal Institute of Chemists and the British Medical Association. The Secretary of State appoints the Chairman, and members hold office for three years. A quorum of the Board is eleven.

The Poisons List

Section 2 of the Act confirms the existence of the Poisons List, and provides that the Secretary of State may, after consultation with the Poisons Board, amend the list by Order. The list is divided into two parts – Part I and Part II. All poisons may be sold by someone lawfully conducting a retail pharmacy business, but Part II poisons may also be sold by persons entered on a Local Authority list. With certain exceptions no other persons may sell non-medicinal poisons.

Section 2(4) directs that in dividing substances between Parts I and II notice shall be taken of the likely use of, and general need of the public to have, such poisons. The present list is contained in the Poisons List Order 1978 (SI 1978 No 2) and it will be seen that Part I poisons contain deadly substances with limited general utility, such as arsenic, cyanide, yellow phosphorus and strychnine, and Part II includes poisons such as formaldehyde, formic, hydrochloric, nitric and sulphuric acids which, while still very hazardous, have somewhat wider use.

As mentioned earlier, if the Secretary of State intends to amend the Poisons List without the Poisons Board's concurrence he must place the proposed Order before each House of Parliament together with his reasons for wishing to proceed.

The Sale of Listed Poisons

Section 3 makes it unlawful for anyone to sell a non-medicinal poison on Part I or II of the Poisons List unless he is lawfully conducting a retail pharmacy business, the sale is made on premises that are a registered pharmacy, and is made under the supervision of a pharmacist. (The definition of a retail pharmacy business and a registered pharmacy are discussed in chapter 7 on the Medicines Act page 71). Sales of a Part II poison are also lawful if made by someone whose name is entered on a Local Authority list in respect of premises on which the sale is made.

The formal requirements of the *Act itself* in respect to the sale of listed poisons are given below but it is important to understand that the Poisons Rules modify these provisions both by extending their application and by relaxing them. Details of the Poisons Rules are given in the next chapter (page 40).

a) Formal requirements for the sale of a poison

Even when made from approved premises by an approved person the sale of a listed poison will still be unlawful unless:

(i) the container is labelled with the name of the poison, its proportion if in a mixture, the word 'POISON' and the name of the seller and the address of his premises,

(ii) (for Part I poisons only) the buyer is a person to whom the poison may be properly sold to the knowledge of the seller or certified as such under the Poisons Rules (see page 41),

(iii) (for Part I poisons only) the seller has recorded in a book kept for the purpose the date of the sale, the name and address of the buyer, the nature and quantity of the poison sold, and the purpose for which the poison is required. The purchaser must sign the book.

The Poisons Rules modify these requirements somewhat (page 40).

b) Exceptions

None of the above requirements applies to the following:

(i) Wholesale dealing,

(ii) exports,

(iii) sales to doctors, dentists and veterinarians for professional use,

(iv) sale for use in connection with a hospital, infirmary, dispensary or other similar institution,

(v) sales by a poisons seller either wholesale or to a purchaser who requires the poisons for his trade or profession, or to comply with a statutory requirement, or to use in a scientific, educational or research institution or if an officer of the Crown for use in the public service.

Again the Poisons Rules modify these requirements somewhat (page 40).

Thus it can be seen that the Act aims to limit the sale of listed poisons to the general public rather than interfere with their availability to trade and professional users.

c) Local authority lists

Section 5 requires local authorities to keep a list of people entitled to sell Part II poisons and of the premises from which such sales may be made. Anyone may apply to have his or her name put on the list. The local authority may refuse to do so, or remove a name already listed, only for failure to pay the prescribed fees or if there is sufficient reason relating to the applicant personally or to his premises to make him unsuitable to be on the list.

A person aggrieved by the refusal of a local authority to list his name or premises may appeal to the Crown Court or in Scotland to the Sheriff. If someone whose name is on the list is convicted of an offence, the court, if it considers the person unfit to have his name on the list, may as part of the sentence disqualify him. This applies to any offence and not just an offence against the Act or the Rules.

Section 6 requires the local authority list to include particulars of the premises in respect of which a person's name is entered, and the list must be open at all reasonable times to inspection by anyone without charge.

d) Penalties

It is an offence to contravene any provision of the Poisons Act or any regulation made thereunder. Section 8 provides that on summary conviction for such an offence a person is liable to a fine not exceeding £50 and if the offence continues after conviction that person is liable to a further fine not exceeding £10 for each day it continues.

Where the offence involves sale, or exposure for sale, of a non-medicinal poison by an employee, it is no defence that the employee acted without the authority of his employer, and any material facts known by the employee are deemed to have been known by the employer.

Poison Rules

Section 7 permits the Secretary of State to make rules known as the Poison Rules to control a variety of activities in respect to poisons. The Rules are to be made on the advice of, or after consultation with, the Poisons Board and may cover any or every non-medicinal poison. The Secretary of State also has the power to revoke any direction he may have previously made.

The rules are contained in the Poisons Rules 1978 (SI 1978 No 1) and will be dealt with in the next chapter (page 40). However, section 7 of the Act provides that rules may be made in respect of the following:

a. Retail, wholesale or supply of non-medicinal poisons whether by restricting their availability or dispensing with the restrictions imposed by the Act,

b. storage, transport and labelling,

c. containers in which non-medicinal poisons may be sold or supplied,

d. the addition of distinguishing substances to non-medicinal poisons,

e. supply or compounding of poisons on a practitioner's prescription,

f. keeping of books,

g. certification of persons who may obtain poisons.

Inspection and Enforcement

To enforce the various requirements of the Act and the Regulations, section 9 establishes a system of inspection that is in part the responsibility of the Pharmaceutical Society of Great Britain and in part that of the local authority.

Pharmaceutical Society inspection

A duty is imposed on the Society to take all reasonable steps by means of inspection and otherwise to secure compliance by pharmacists and persons carrying on a retail pharmacy business with the provisions of the Act and the Rules. To do so the Society must appoint such number of inspectors as is approved by the Privy Council. An inspector, whose appointment is subject to approval by the Privy Council, must be a pharamacist. His terms and conditions of service are determined by the Council of the Pharmaceutical Society subject to approval by the Privy Council.

When acting in the course of his duties as such an inspector has a power of entry to any registered pharmacy or, in the case of Part I poisons, other premises on which he reasonably believes a breach of the law has been committed. In either case he may make such examination and enquiry and take such samples (subject to payment for them) as are necessary to determine whether the provisions of the Act or the Rules have been complied with.

Local authority inspectors

Every local authority has a duty by means of inspection and otherwise to take all reasonable steps to secure compliance with the Act and its Rules by persons selling Part II poisons who are not conducting a retail pharmacy business and, in respect of Part I and Part II poisons, compliance by people who are conducting a lawful retail pharmacy business in so far as the business is carried out at premises that are not a registered pharmacy. To do so the local authority must appoint inspectors and, with the agreement of the Pharmaceutical Society, one of the Society's inspectors may also be a local authority inspector. Local authority inspectors have a power of entry at all reasonable times on any premises on the local authority list, or any other premises where the inspector has reasonable suspicion that a breach of the law in respect of Part II poisons has been committed. In each case he may make such examination and enquiry and take such samples (for which he must pay) as are necessary to investigate the suspected breach. A local authority inspector has the power to initiate proceedings under the Act with the consent of the local authority and may conduct such a case in court, although he is not a solicitor or barrister.

Wilfully obstructing an inspector, refusing to supply him with a sample or failing to give information is an offence liable on summary conviction to a fine not exceeding £5.

Chapter Five

Poisons Rules 1978 : Practical Aspects

Introduction

There has always been a degree of confusion about the Poisons List and Rules under the Pharmacy and Poisons Act 1933. To some extent this has been due to the large number of parts to the Poisons List and schedules to the Rules. Now that the 1972 Poisons Act deals only with non-medicinal poisons the situation is somewhat clearer. The present Poisons Rules (SI 1978 No. 1) contains 29 paragraphs and 15 schedules and, while still complex, is clearer than earlier versions.

The poisons law has only limited applications to the Health Services, the main use of poisons being in the public health sector. Although they will be dealt with relatively briefly in this book they are nevertheless of interest, for they illustrate on the one hand the extent to which a Minister of the Crown may in effect alter the provisions of a Statute by delegated legislation and on the other how a balance is struck (or attempted) between the need to protect the public from the hazards of poisons and the needs of industrial firms etc. which have legitimate uses for such substances.

The Poisons Rules are divided into five broad parts: those modifying the application of the Act itself, those that impose extra restrictions on the sale of poisons, those that deal with labelling and containers, those that deal with storage and transport and those that deal with records and documentation. The Rules will now be considered under these broad heads.

Modification of the Act (Rules 3 - 6)

Before considering these rules we should recapitulate the particular provisions of the Act affected. Section 3(1)(a) limits the lawful sale of a Part I poison to a person conducting a retail pharmacy business when the sale is made from a registered pharmacy and under the supervision of a pharmacist. Section 3(1)(b) provides that a Part II poison may only be sold lawfully by a retail pharmacy business as above or by someone on the local authority list from premises in respect of which the listing is made. Section 3(1)(c) requires the poison sold to be labelled in the prescribed way and to include the name and address of the seller. Section 3(2) requires a purchaser of Part I poisons to be certified as, or known to the seller as, a person to whom poisons may properly be sold, and at each sale an entry in the poisons book must be made and signed by the purchaser. Section 4 provides that the provisions of Sections 3(1) and 3(2) do not extend to wholesale dealing, exports, sales to practitioners, sales to hospitals and similar institutions or sales to a person carrying on a business in which poisons are regularly sold or used. Rules 3 - 8 modify the application of Sections 3 and 4 as follows:

Shopkeepers (Rule 3)

A shopkeeper may not sell poisons from premises connected with his retail business even though the sale is exempt by Section 4, unless he complies with Section 3(1)(a) or (b) as the case may be.

Labelling (Rule 4)

The labelling requirements of Section 3(1)(c) and of Rules 15 - 20 (see page 44) are to apply also to sales exempted by Section 4 (but not to exports) and also to the supply of poisons other than those on sale. However, these labelling requirements (except the need to put on to the container/label the name and address of the seller and, if a liquid, the words 'not to be taken' – Rule 19) do not apply to the sale or supply of a poison included in Schedule 2 to the Rules to someone who carries on a business in which poisons are sold wholesale or who uses poisons in the manufacture of other articles and requires them for that purpose. Schedule 2 includes the commoner industrial chemicals such as ammonia, formaldehyde, a range of acids and alkalis and yellow phosphorus.

Purchasers (Rule 5)

The provisions of Section 3(2), concerning to whom poisons may be sold and the formalities of the sale, which in the Act itself apply only to Part I poisons are made by Rule 5 to apply only to poisons in Schedule 1 to the Rules, whether they be Part I or Part II poisons, but not to anything else. Many of the Schedule 1 poisons are contained in Part II of the Poisons List and the effect of this rule is to bring many Part II poisons under the provisions of Section 3(2). However, nicotine for use in agricultural and horticultural insecticides in concentrations of not more than 4% w/w is exempted by Schedule 13.

Extension of Section 3(2) (Rule 6)
Section 3(2) of the Act, concerning purchasers and the form of the sale as modified by Rule 5 above, is made by Rule 6 to apply to sales exempted by Section 4 (except exports) and also to commercial samples. However, these provisions do not apply to manufacturers and wholesale dealers if the poison is sold or supplied to someone whose business is selling poisons or who regularly uses poisons in the course of manufacturing other articles.

Where a sale of a poison is for the purpose of a trade or profession an entry in the poisons book is not required provided the seller obtains before the sale a written order signed by the purchaser and including his name and address, trade etc, details of the poison, the quantity and its proposed use. An entry in the poison book of 'signed order' is to be made with a reference number by which the original order can be identified.

Rule 6 also makes provision for the emergency supply of a poison with the poison book formalities to be completed within 24 hours.

Exemptions (Rules 7 and 8)
Rule 7 exempts barium carbonate and zinc phosphide preparations for use as rat and mice killers from the provisions of the Act and Rules as they apply to Schedule 1 poisons. Rule 8 exempts from all provisions of the Act and the Rules substances in groups I and II of Schedule 3 to the Rules.

Group I includes such common substances as adhesives, enamels, fireworks, matches, motor fuel, photographic paper, rubber and varnish. Group II includes a wide variety of substances for specific uses or in specific concentrations, for example, arsenic in certain chemical forms in reagent kits, barium salts or bromomethane in fire extinguishers, formaldehyde in less than 5% w/w concentration, mercuric chloride as a dressing for seeds or bulbs, and sulphuric acid of less than 9% w/w concentration in car batteries etc.

Further Restrictions on Poisons Sales (Rules 9 - 14)

Retail Pharmacy Business (Rule 9)
All sales from a retail pharmacy of Schedule 1 poisons must be made by, or under the supervision of, a pharmacist even though the poison is in Part II of the Poisons List.

Listed Sellers (Rule 10)
Rule 10 provides that a shopkeeper who is a listed seller of Part II poisons must:

(i) sell all poisons (except ammonia, hydrochloric, nitric and sulphuric acids, and potassium quadroxalate) in a closed container closed by the manufacturer from whom he obtained it – ie he is not permitted to dispense his sales from a larger stock.

(ii) himself effect the sale of a poison if it is in Schedule 1. Alternatively, the sale may be made by a responsible deputy whose name is included on the seller's application for a local authority listing.

Rule 10 goes on to restrict the sales of poisons in Schedule 4, as far as listed Part II sellers are concerned, as follows:

(i) Poisons in Part A of Schedule 4 may not be sold by a listed seller except for the uses indicated in that Schedule and then, in addition to the standard labelling provisions, the poison must be clearly labelled with the specific use and a warning that it is to be used only for that purpose. Part A of Schedule 4 contains a wide variety of chemicals used in agriculture, horticulture and forestry.

(ii) Poisons in Part B of Schedule 4 may be sold by listed Part II sellers only to purchasers whose trade or business is agriculture, horticulture or forestry, and where the poison is to be used for any of those purposes. Part B of Schedule 4 contains a wide range of substances which are used in agriculture, horticulture and forestry but which are more dangerous than those in Part A and therefore limited to professional users.

(iii) Cycloheximide may not be sold by a listed Part II seller unless the purchaser is engaged in the trade of forestry and requires it for that purpose.

Colouring of certain poisons (Rule 11)
Poisons listed in Schedule 14 (mainly phosphorus compounds) which are to be used as weedkillers or to treat or prevent infestation by animals or plants must have added to them a dye to render them a distinctive colour. The requirement, which is aimed at visual identification of these poisons, applies both to liquids and solid preparations of Schedule 14 poisons. It does not apply if the poisons are themselves a distinctive colour or are for export.

Wholesale sales to shopkeepers (Rule 12)
A wholesaler may not sell a Part I poison to a shopkeeper unless he is conducting a retail pharmacy business or the purchaser has declared in writing that he does not intend to sell the poison on any premises used in connection with his retail business.

Specific restrictions on certain poisons (Rules 13 and 14)
Except for export sales, wholesale sales and sales to a person or institution concerned with scientific education, research or chemical analysis, the sale or supply of the following poisons is unlawful except as indicated below:

(i) *Strychnine* – Sale permitted only to persons with written authority from Ministry of Agriculture, Fisheries and Food for the purpose of killing moles, or to an Officer of the same Ministry with written authority for the purpose of killing foxes in connection with a rabies control order.

(ii) *Fluoroacetic acid and fluoroacetamide* – Sale permitted only to a person certified by the appropriate officer of a local authority or a port health authority for use as a rodenticide by the authority's employees in ships, sewers, drains and warehouses.

(iii) *Thallium salts* – Sales permitted only to local or port authority in exercise of their statutory duty, a government department or officer of the Crown for the public service or a person duly authorised by the Ministry of Agriculture, Fisheries and Food for killing mice, rats and moles in the course of a business of pest control, or to a business using thallium salts for manufacturing other articles.

(iv) *Zinc phosphide* – Sales permitted only to a local authority to exercise its statutory power or to a government department or officer of the Crown in the public service or for the purposes of a trade or business.

(v) *Sodium and potassium arsenites* – No permitted sales except for export, wholesale or for scientific, educational, research or analytical purposes.

(vi) *Calcium, sodium and potassium cyanide* – Only sales permitted are those exempt from control by Section 4 of the Act.

Labelling and Containers

Labelling

Rules 15 - 20 deal in detail with the labelling of poisons.

Rule 15 requires the prescribed labelling to be in a conspicuous and unobscured position on every container and outer pack. There is, however, no need to label a transparent outer pack or a covering used solely for transport or delivery.

Rule 16 requires the name of the poison to be that given in the Poisons List or, if the list uses a group term, then the accepted scientific name. For the substances listed in Schedule 5 the name of the poison may be expressed as indicated in that schedule. Thus, for arsenic compounds the labelling may refer to the contents as arsenic trioxide or pentoxide in the proportion that the material would yield if converted to one of these substances. This is in line with analytical practice.

Rule 17 requires the label to state what proportion of the contents are the said poison and, in the case of Schedule 5, substances that may be expressed as a standard equivalent. Where the proportion is expressed as a percentage the label must show if this is calculated weight for weight, volume for volume or weight for volume.

Rule 18 requires that substances in Schedule 6 are not to bear the word 'poison' but the special wording indicated by this schedule. The prescribed wording brings to the attention of the user the special hazards of the substance. Thus, for hair dyes containing alkylated benzene diamines the label must read: "Caution – This preparation may cause serious inflammation of the skin in certain persons and should be used only in accordance with expert advice." Whether the word 'poison' or the special Schedule 6 wording is to be used if the substance is a Schedule 1 poison the wording must be in red or on a red background. In all cases the prescribed words must be on a separate label or surrounded by a line separating them from all other wording.

Rule 19 requires liquid poisons of capacity of not more than three litres to be labelled 'Not to be taken'.

Rule 20 deals with the name and address of the seller/supplier on the label. It provides that for sales from a depot or warehouse the name and address of the supplier's principal place of business or, if a registered company, his registered office are acceptable.

Containers (Rule 21)
It is unlawful to sell or supply any poison unless it is in an impervious container sufficiently stout to prevent leakage as a result of ordinary handling. If it is a liquid supplied in a bottle of not more than 1.14 litres the outer surface of the bottle must be fluted or ribbed to make it recognisable by touch. However, this latter requirement does not apply to exports or sales for scientific, educational and research use.

The Packaging and Labelling of Dangerous Substances Regulations 1978
The Packaging and Labelling of Dangerous Substances Regulations 1978 (SI 1978 No. 209) implements an EEC directive (67/548/EEC and 76/907/EEC) on the classification, packaging and labelling of dangerous substances. These regulations lay down requirements for the packaging and labelling of those dangerous substances listed in Schedule 1. Together with S3(1)(c) of the Poisons Act 1972 and the Poisons Rules 1978 they would impose dual packaging and labelling

requirements on substances covered by both the Regulations and the Poisons Act: In order to avoid this the Poisons (Amendment) Rules 1978 (SI 1978 No. 672) provides that as far as poisons that are listed in Schedule 1 to the Packaging and Labelling of Dangerous Substances Regulations are concerned they are relieved from the requirements of sub paragraphs (i) to (iii) of Section 3(1)(c) of the Poisons Act and Rules 15 - 18, 19(1) and (3), 20(1) and (2), 21, 22(1), 23 and 24(1). They are also relieved from the requirement of S3(1)(c)(iv) of the Act and Rule 20(3) and (4) (recording the name and address of the sale of a poison) except in the case of a poison sold retail by a shopkeeper.

One of the effects of this amendment will be to release manufacturers and others from the legal requirement to pack certain substances in fluted or ribbed bottles. However a Home Office press notice expresses the hope that fluted bottles will continue to be used in the interests of safety of the blind and partially sighted.

Requirements of the Packaging and Labelling of Dangerous Substances Regulations

The Regulations apply to "prescribed dangerous substances" which are those substances listed in Schedule 1. However, substances which are medicinal products as defined by S130 of the Medicines Act or have been brought under its control by the application of S104 or S105, motor fuels, munitions, pesticides, compressed or liquified gases, paraffin and substances delivered by pipeline or into a storage tank are exempt.

Containers

Regulation 4 requires the container to be designed, constructed and secured to prevent escape of the contents under normal handling conditions. The container must be constructed of a material that will not be attacked by the contents.

Labelling

Regulation 5 requires the container to be labelled with the name of the substance as indicated in Schedule 1 together with the name and address of the manufacturer, importer, wholesaler or supplier. The general risk associated with the product as indicated in column 2 of Schedule 1 must be shown by use of the appropriate symbol, for example, a skull and crossbones for 'toxic', a picture of a flame for 'highly inflammable'. The particular risk is to be indicated by the wording indicated by Schedule 1 column 3 and Schedule 3, while the safety precautions required are to be indicated (Schedule 1 column 4 and Schedule 4).

Regulation 6 requires the marking on containers to be indelible, easily read and specific dimensions for labels and symbols used.

The Regulations are made under S2 of the European Communities Act 1972, and are enforced as if they were a health and safety regulation made under S15 of the Health & Safety at Work etc. Act 1974. Where a prescribed dangerous substance is supplied from premises registered under S75 of the Medicines Act 1968 (ie a registered pharmacy) the enforcing authority is the Pharmaceutical Society of Great Britain.

Storage and Transport of Poisons. The Poisons Rules.

Storage (Rule 22)

Poisons must be stored in impervious containers sufficiently stout to prevent damage from ordinary handling. Schedule 1 poisons at a retail shop must be stored in a cupboard or drawer reserved for the purpose, or in a separate part of the premises to which the public do not have access, or on a shelf reserved for poisons (but food, and beverages, must not be stored under that shelf).

Agricultural, horticultural and forestry poisons must also be stored away from food.

Transport (Rules 23 and 24)

It is unlawful to consign poisons for transport unless they are stoutly packed to prevent leakage. For poisons in Schedule 7 the outside of the container in which the poison is being transported must be conspicuously labelled with the name of the poison and a notice to keep it separate from food or empty food containers. Poisons must not be transported in the same vehicle as food unless they are in a separated part.

Documentation

Rules 25 - 29 are concerned with documentation in various forms.

Local authority lists (Rule 25)

Schedule 9 to the Rules outlines the form in which the local authority list must be kept, and Rule 25 states the various fees to be paid in respect of entries on the list. Schedule 8 outlines the form in which an application for inclusion on the list must be made.

Certificates (Rule 26)

The form of a document certifying that a person may be properly sold a poison (as required by S3(2)(a)) is given in Schedule 10. Rule 26 provides that all householders may give such a certificate. If the householder giving the certificate is not known to the seller then the certificate must be endorsed by a police officer in charge of a police station.

Records (Rules 27 and 28)
Rule 27 requires that poisons books be kept in the form laid out in Schedule 11. Rule 28 requires such books to be kept for two years from the date of the last entry.

In order to assist the reader to review the Poisons Rules, two tables are given below. Table 1 gives a summary of the main Rules, while Table 2 gives a summary of the main Schedules to the Rules.

Table 1 Summary of main Poisons Rules

Rule 3	deals with sales by shopkeepers.
Rule 4	extends (with exceptions) labelling requirements to sales exempt under S4 of the Act.
Rule 5	Provisions of S3(2) of Act to apply to poisons in Schedule 1 whether or not they are in Part I of the List.
Rule 6	Provisions of S3(2) of Act and Rule 5 above to apply to sales exempted by S4. Also deals with emergency supply of poisons.
Rule 7	Exempts barium carbonate and zinc phosphide rat and mice killer from controls imposed on Schedule 1 poisons.
Rule 8	Exempts from all control of Act and Rules substances in Schedule 3.
Rule 9	All poison sales (Part I and II) from retail pharmacies to be made under supervision of pharmacist.
Rule 10	Lays down rules for sales by listed seller.
Rule 11	Requires certain poisons in Schedule 14 to be coloured.
Rule 12	Wholesaler may only sell Part I poisons to retail pharmacy.
Rule 13 and 14	Prohibits all sales of certain poisons to the public with exceptions.
Rule 15, 16, 17, 19, 20	Deals with labelling poisons.
Rule 18	Requires special labelling for substances in Schedule 6.

Rule 21	Deals with poisons containers including need for fluted bottles.
Rule 22	Deals with storage of poisons.
Rule 23	Deals with transport of poisons.
Rule 24	Special transport requirements for Schedule 7 poisons.
Rule 25	Deals with local authority lists.
Rule 26	Deals with certificates.
Rule 27 and 28	Deals with records.

Table 2 Summary of main Schedules to Poisons Rules 1978

Schedule 1	List of poisons to which special rules apply unless exempted by Rule 7.
Schedule 2	List of poisons exempted from labelling requirements in certain circumstances.
Schedule 3	List of poisons totally exempt from Act and Rules in certain circumstances.
Schedule 4 Part A	Lists the only forms in which certain poisons may be sold by listed sellers of Part II poisons.
Part B	List of poisons that may only be sold to people engaged in trade or business of agriculture, horticulture, or forestry, for use in that trade or profession, by a listed Part II seller.
Schedule 5	How to express the proportion of certain poisons in substances containing them.
Schedule 6	Specific wording required on labels on certain poisons.
Schedule 7	List of poisons to be specially labelled for transport.
Schedule 14	List of poisons which must be coloured in certain circumstances.

Chapter Six

MEDICINES ACT 1968

Controls on Medicinal Products

Introduction and Legal History

We have already seen that the law relating to dangerous drugs and poisons developed late in legal history. However, as far as medicinal substances are concerned, it was not until 1968 that there was any comprehensive system of legislation controlling their manufacture, sale and supply.

If a medicinal product happened also to be a drug of addiction it would be controlled by the dangerous drugs legislation, at least from the 1920s. Similarly, if it was a listed poison, it would have been controlled by the contemporary poisons legislation. The Pharmacy and Poisons Act 1933 contained in Schedule 4 a category of 'prescription only' poisons. This was used to some extent to control newly introduced medicines which were often put into Schedule 4, not because they were toxic but because that together with the Therapeutic Substances Acts was the only way in which their availability could be controlled. Thus the only control on the availability of barbiturates up to 1978 was that provided by Schedule 4.

In 1875 the first Food and Drugs Act was passed which prohibited the adulteration of food and drugs, and provided standards for them. However, these Acts (the 1955 Food and Drugs Act is the most recent) were only of limited application to medicines, partly because most drugs were originally of vegetable origin for which no satisfactory analytical standard existed and also because there was no need for a manufacturer of a proprietary medicine to declare its composition provided he paid the appropriate duty on his product under the Medicine Stamp Acts. In 1941 the Pharmacy and Medicines Act required that the composition of a medicine should be declared and abolished the stamp duty.

Another series of Acts partially controlled one particular type of medicinal product. The Therapeutic Substances Act 1925 controlled the manufacture (but not sale or supply) of substances that were not capable of chemical analysis. These were mainly vaccines, sera and antitoxins, and as antibiotics made their appearance these were also included in its provisions. However, the Therapeutic Substances Acts 1925-56 assumed that the substances they controlled were not dangerous by nature and thus initially they did not control their supply. With the advent of penicillin it was clear that the availability of this substance should be limited. The Therapeutic Substances Act could not provide the restriction and penicillin could hardly be called a Schedule 4 poison. For this reason the Penicillin Act 1947 and the Therapeutic Substances (Prevention of Misuse) Act 1953 were passed to limit the availability of antibiotics to the public to those available from a doctor's prescription only.

Thus, as late as the 1960's, anyone could manufacture and wholesale medicines without any control whatsoever provided they were not a TSA substance, a listed poison or a dangerous drug. The total unacceptability of this state of affairs in a modern society was demonstrated to the public by the thalidomide tragedy. In 1959 a working party was set up by the Government to consider the need for new controls. In 1963 the Ministry of Health issued a series of papers outlining the form they considered new legislation should take and these were circulated to interested parties. In 1967 a White Paper entitled 'Forthcoming Legislation on the Safety, Quality and Description of Drugs and Medicines' (Cmnd 3395) was published and on 25th October 1968 the Medicines Act received the Royal Assent. However, it was not until 1978 that most of this Act was brought into force. Thus it had taken almost 20 years to establish the comprehensive set of medicines controls that now exist.

Medicines Act 1968

Introduction

The Medicines Act covers both human and animal medicines and medicated animal feedstuffs, but for the purposes of this book only the human aspects will be covered. The Act repeals the 1933 Pharmacy and Poisons Act and the Therapeutic Substances Act 1956 and extends to Scotland and Northern Ireland. Of the three modern statutes in this area of law (the other two being the Misuse of Drugs Act 1971 and the Poisons Act 1972) the Medicines Act is by far the largest. The Act contains eight parts, 136 sections and eight schedules and covers some 165 pages. Up to the beginning of 1980 some 140 Statutory Instruments had been made under the Act. The Act is comprehensive. It covers virtually every possible activity concerned with a medicinal product and also some related areas such as retail pharmacies and the British Pharmacopoeia. Broadly speaking, the Act may be considered under seven broad heads – the administrative system, the licensing system, the sale and supply of medicines to the public, retail pharmacies, the packing and labelling of medicinal products, the promotion of medicines, and the British Pharmacopoeia. In this chapter the administrative and licensing systems will be considered while in the next (chapter 7) the provisions of the Act in respect of retail sale, promotion, retail pharmacies, packing and labelling and the British Pharmacopoeia will be covered.

Definition of medicinal product

The Act controls 'medicinal products' and these are defined by Section 130. A medicinal product is 'any substance or article (not being an instrument, apparatus or appliance) which is manufactured, sold, supplied, imported or exported for use wholly or mainly for administration to human beings or animals for a medicinal purpose or as an ingredient used in a pharmacy or hospital, or by a practitioner, or by a retail herbal remedy business in the preparation of a substance to be administered to humans or animals for a medicinal purpose.'

Section 130 defines a medicinal purpose as: the treatment or prevention of disease, the diagnosis of a disease, of physiological states, contraception, the induction of anaesthesia or the prevention of, or interference with, any physiological function. The Act excludes from the definition of a medicinal product a substance manufactured for administration to humans or animals to test what action it has, dental filling substances and bandages and dressings except where they are used to apply a medicament. However, these exclusions may be restricted by an order made by the Minister of Health or Minister of Agriculture, and such orders have already been made for dental filling substances and certain surgical materials which are now covered by some of the provisions of the Act.

Section 130 permits the Minister of Health (or Agriculture) to define substances and articles that are not to be treated as medicinal products, but by Section 104 they can extend the Act to non-medicinal products if they are made solely or mainly for a medicinal use (for example, surgical sutures) or (S105) to any substance that is used as an ingredient in the manufacture of a medicine or a substance capable of causing danger to the health of the community if used without proper safeguards. Orders under S104 and 105 may specify which parts of the Act are to apply.

Thus, in order to determine whether or not a substance is a medicinal product, it is necessary not only to refer to the Act itself but also to the body of statutory instruments made under the Act to date.

The Administrative System

It is inevitable that a complex and comprehensive measure such as the Medicines Act 1968 will require a complex administrative system for its operation. The Act itself cannot be fully understood without a knowledge of this administrative system while, to a lesser extent, the administrative system cannot be understood without an understanding of the substantive parts of the Act. In applying the provisions of the Act a variety of bodies are involved and these are summarised here:

The Ministers

The Act imposes a variety of functions on the 'ministers', or the 'health ministers', or the 'agriculture ministers', or the 'appropriate ministers'. Section 1 defines the health ministers as the Minister of Health, the Secretary of State concerned with health in Scotland and the Minister of Health and Social Services in Northern Ireland acting jointly. Similarly, the term, 'the agriculture ministers', means the Minister of Agriculture, Fisheries and Food, the Secretary of State concerned with agriculture in Scotland and the Minister of Agriculture in Northern Ireland acting jointly. The term, 'the ministers', means all of these ministers acting jointly. The term, the 'appropriate ministers', for any function where veterinary drugs and the treatment of animals are not involved means the Health Ministers and in any other case means all of the ministers.

The licensing authority

As will be seen later, the Act controls many dealings with medicinal products by means of licences (see page 56) and the authority that grants, renews, varies, suspends or revokes a licence is called the licensing authority. Section 6 provides that this authority is a body consisting of all of the ministers. However, where the Act requires the licensing authority to fulfil a particular function it may be done by any one minister acting alone or by two or more acting jointly, and the term licensing authority is to be interpreted in this way.

The Medicines Commission

Section 2 establishes a body called the Medicines Commission as a body corporate with perpetual succession and a common seal and provides that its members are disqualified from membership of the House of Commons under the House of Commons Disqualification Act 1975. There are to be not less than eight members of the Commission to be appointed by the Ministers after consultation with appropriate organisations. There must be at least one person with wide and recent experience of each of the following: the practice of medicine, veterinary medicine, pharmacy, chemistry (other than pharmaceutical chemistry) and the pharmaceutical industry. There were 19 members listed in the Commission's annual report for 1978. The Ministers are to appoint one member of the Commission as chairman.

The general functions of the Commission are outlined in Section 3 of the Act. The Commission is to advise the Ministers in relation to the operation of the Act and the exercise of any powers granted them under it. The advice is to be given both when the Commission is consulted and when it thinks fit to do so. The Commission must also make recommendations to the Ministers about the number, function and membership of any committees that are created under Section 4 of the Act (see below). From time to time it must review these committees and make whatever recommendations for change it thinks appropriate.

Medicines Act committees

Section 4 of the Act empowers the Ministers to establish one or more committees connected with the execution of the Act or in support of their powers under it. In particular the Section provides that committees may be set up to give advice on the safety, quality and efficacy of medicinal products, to collect information on adverse reactions to medicinal products, and to administer the British Pharmacopoeia (see page 73).

Up to 1979 five committees had been set up:

The Committee on Safety of Medicines (CSM) (SI 1970 Nos. 746 and 1257)

This committee was set up to give advice on the safety, quality and efficacy of human medicines and to promote the collection and investigation of adverse reactions. In its 1978 annual report the CSM listed six sub-committees – one on adverse reactions, one on chemistry, pharmacy and standards, one on 'biologicals', one on standards for herbal remedies, one on toxicity, clinical trials and therapeutic efficacy, and a joint sub-committee on anti-microbial substances (with the Veterinary Products Committee).

Veterinary Products Committee (VPC) (SI 1970 No. 1304)

The remit of this committee is to give advice on the safety, quality and efficacy of veterinary products and to collect and investigate adverse reactions. It has one sub-committee – the feedstuffs sub-committee.

British Pharmacopoeia Commission (SI 1970 No. 1256)

This is the body set up to administer all aspects of the British Pharmacopoeia (see page 73). At present it has 22 different committees.

Committee on the Review of Medicines (SI 1975 No. 1006)
This committee was set up to review the safety, quality and efficacy of all human medicines for which a product licence has been issued (see page 59) and to advise the licensing authority. The committee is reviewing categories of medicinal products in turn and making general recommendations while the CSM essentially deals with each medicinal product in isolation. In its 1978 annual report the CRM had four sub-committees – one on anti-rheumatic agents, one on analgesics, one on psychotropic drugs and one on immunological products.

Committee on Dental and Surgical Materials (SI 1975 No. 1473)
This committee is to give advice on the safety, efficacy and quality of animal and human uses of substances, articles, instruments, apparatus and appliances to which the Act applies but which are outside the remit of the CSM or the VPC. It is also required to promote the collection of information on adverse reactions. The committee is at present dealing with such things as intra-uterine contraceptive devices, bone cements, surgical sutures and absorbable dressings.

General Provisions for the Medicines Commission and the Section 4 Committees
Section 5 and Schedule 1 to the Act and SI 1970 No. 746 lay down a variety of provisions for the Medicines Commission and the section 4 committees. Thus the Commission and each committee must prepare an annual report to be presented jointly by the Ministers to Parliament. The Commission and Committees are to be provided with such staff and accommodation as appear necessary to the Ministers. The Ministers may pay them remuneration (if any) and allowances subject to Treasury consent. It is laid down that the Commission and the committees and the sub-committees are not agents of the Crown and do not enjoy Crown immunity.

The Medicines Division: Enforcement: The Pharmaceutical Society
The part of the Department of Health and Social Security which is responsible for the Medicines Act is the Medicines Division. That Division is responsible for licensing, enforcement and inspection under the Act, for preparing new legislation (which in effect means Statutory instruments), for international relations on medicines (particularly with the EEC) and for providing a body of professional civil servants to support the Commission and the committees. Of these functions, those of enforcement and inspection must be considered a little further.

The duty to enforce the provisions of the Act and any regulations made under it falls to the appropriate Minister in England or Wales (S108), Scotland (S109) and Northern Ireland (S110). To fulfil their duty the Ministers may delegate many functions to other authorities, but the licensing provisions and any relating to the premises of hospitals or practitioners may not be delegated. Delegation may be to the local food and drug authority and/or to the Pharmaceutical Society, and Sections 108-110 determine the extent to which such delegation may be made. In order to carry out these functions an enforcement authority (for example, a local food and drug authority, the Pharmaceutical Society or the Medicines Division itself) may appoint inspectors. Section 111 gives such inspectors wide-ranging rights of entry including entry to a private house if 24 hours' notice is given or earlier under the authority of a magistrate's warrant. Section 112 gives inspectors a power to take samples and seize goods and documents and S113 lays down the procedure for taking such samples including the splitting of it into three parts, one to be returned to the manufacturer or seller. Section 114 makes it an offence to obstruct an inspector in a variety of ways. Section 118 prohibits an inspector from disclosing information obtained in the course of his duty except in the performance of that duty, while S119 provides that, where he honestly believes he is acting in the course of his duty, he is not *personally* liable for his acts.

The Licensing System

A wide variety of dealings with medicinal products is controlled by a licensing system and Part II of the Medicines Act (SS 6-50) deals with this. We have already seen that the licensing authority is in effect one or more Ministers (S6).

The need for a licence

Section 7 provides that, subject to certain exceptions considered below, no-one in the course of a business carried on by him may sell, supply or export any medicinal product, or procure the same, or procure the manufacture or assembly of a medicinal product for these purposes, or import any medicinal product unless in accordance with a licence issued for the purpose. Such a licence is called a *product licence*. A product licence for a medicinal product other than an imported one is required only by the person responsible in the course of a business for its composition, and that in effect means either the person who manufactures the product or to whose order it is manufactured.

Section 8 provides that, subject to certain exceptions (below), no-one shall in the course of a business carried on by him manufacture or assemble a medicinal product, or sell or offer to sell wholesale any medicinal product except in accordance with a licence issued for the purpose. In the first case a *manufacturer's licence* is required while in the second a *wholesale dealer's licence* is needed.

Exemptions from the need for a licence

Practitioners

Doctors, dentists and veterinarians are exempted the licensing requirements by S9. A doctor or dentist may prepare or import, or order the preparation or importation of, any medicinal product, or manufacture, assemble, sell or supply, or procure the same for administration to a particular patient of his. This exemption extends to a practitioner acting on the order of another. However, regulations provide that a doctor may not hold in stock more than 5 litres of a liquid preparation or 2.5 kg of a solid substance. It should be noted that this provision envisages a 'particular patient' and does not give the doctor a wider freedom.

A doctor may approach a pharmaceutical manufacturer to prepare a medicinal product for use by him under this exception. Statutory Instruments 1971 No. 1450 and 1972 No. 1200 provide that the manufacturer need not hold a product licence provided he does not solicit the doctor or advertise such products. However, he must hold a manufacturer's licence that has been extended to include such 'special services' by the licensing authority.

Pharmacists

Section 10 provides that no licence is required for a variety of activities undertaken in a registered pharmacy (see page 72), health centre or hospital provided these are carried out by, or under the supervision of, a pharmacist. The activities are: preparing or dispensing a medicinal product to a practitioner's prescription, assembling a medicinal product or procuring the same. In a registered pharmacy the exception also covers preparing or dispensing a medicinal product to be given to a patient on the pharmacist's own judgement provided the patient is present in the pharmacy at the time. Stocks of medicinal products may be prepared by a pharmacist for this purpose or for use at a hospital or health centre.

As with a practitioner a pharmacist may obtain his exempted supplies from a manufacturer with a 'specials' licence, and that manufacturer does not need a product licence.

Nurses and midwives

Section 11 permits a registered nurse or a certified midwife to assemble a medicinal product without the need for a manufacturer's licence. 'Assembly' is defined by S132 as either enclosing a medicinal product with or without other medicinal products of the same description in a container to be labelled before sale or supply or, if already enclosed, labelled before sale or supply.

Other exemptions

There are a variety of other exceptions from the need for a licence. No licence is required for the sale, supply, manufacture or assembly of any herbal remedy by a herbalist, i.e. someone who, in the course of a business, supplies herbal remedies for treatment on his own judgement (S12). A herbal remedy is defined by S132 as being produced by subjecting plants to drying, crushing or any other process, or a mixture whose sole ingredients are two or more such substances and water or other inert substance.

At the moment no product licence is required to export a medicinal product (S48) although a manufacturer's licence is needed. However, this is only a transitional provision and S48 provides that on an appointed day the product licensing system will be extended to exports.

A medicinal product which has been imported may be re-exported without any form of licence, provided it is not changed in any way (S14). However, these exceptions in relation to exports and re-exports have already been withdrawn in the case of antigens, antitoxins, vaccines, insulin and other substances produced from animals (SI 1971 No. 1198 and 1971 No. 1309).

Licences of right

It was obviously not possible to introduce the full licensing requirements of the 1968 Act without some transitional provisions. Section 25 provided for this need by means of licences of right. Where a medicinal product was effectively on the market before September 1st 1971 a product licence of right could be obtained. Similarly, anyone manufacturing or wholesaling medicinal products for 12 months before the same date could obtain manufacturer's licences or wholesale dealer's licences of right.

Applications for licences of right required considerably less information than is required by the licensing authority for a full licence. No licences of right could be applied for after July 1st 1972, and the safety, quality and efficacy of medicinal products subject to licences of right are being reviewed by the Committee on Review of Medicines. In due course all licences of right will be reviewed and, if satisfactory, will be converted to full licences.

Position of hospitals

Because the Medicines Act does not bind the Crown, National Health Service hospitals are not caught by the licensing system. However, the DHSS has authorised the Medicines Division to inspect all manufacturing units in the NHS and make recommendations. As a result of this procedure several such units have been closed.

Licensing procedure

General

Section 18 requires applications for licences to be made to the licensing authority in the prescribed manner. The licensing authority has the power to grant, refuse, review, suspend, revoke or vary a licence. Section 18 permits the authority to issue a licence subject to such provisions as it thinks fit. However, such provisions may not include a stipulation on the price of the medicine and the authority may not refuse the grant of a licence on the grounds of price. Where the authority intends to refuse a licence on the grounds of safety, quality or efficacy it must consult the appropriate committee – the Committee on Safety of Medicines or the Veterinary Products Committee. If the Committee recommends that a licence should not be granted the applicant must be informed and given the opportunity of appearing before the Committee. If the Committee still refuses to recommend a licence the applicant may then be heard by the Medicines Commission. The final decision is taken by the licensing authority which must take note of the advice of the Committee and the Commission but is not bound to follow it. The applicant is able to contest an adverse decision only on the grounds that it is outside the powers of the Act or that it was arrived at without compliance with the formalities of the Act or the Regulations (S107).

Where the licensing authority refuses a licence on grounds not related to safety, quality or efficacy, or refuses a licence in spite of contrary advice from the Committee or Commission, then the applicant has a right to a hearing before an independent person appointed by the authority.

Section 28 states the grounds upon which the licensing authority may suspend, revoke or vary a licence. These include false statements in an application, failure to observe the provisions of a licence or failure to fulfil, or continue to fulfil, a standard of safety, quality or efficacy.

Product licences

A product licence is required by a person who imports or first sells or supplies a substance after it has become a medicinal product. Thus, this is either the manufacturer, importer or the person who procures the manufacture of the product to his specification. A product licence is required to permit the sale, supply or export of the medicinal product or its manufacture or assembly.

Section 19 requires the licensing authority to consider the safety, quality and efficacy of the medicinal product in considering an application for a product licence. The form and contents of the application are given in SIs 1971 No. 973,

1972 No. 1201, and 1975 No. 681. Extensive details are called for. These include the activities to be licensed, pharmaceutical, physical and chemical details of the product, method of manufacture, assembly and quality control, details of containers and labelling. Considerable details of animal pharmacological and toxicological testing and of human trials are required to establish safety and efficacy.

Standard provisions for all licences are dealt with by S47, and SIs 1971 No. 972, 1972 No. 1226, 1974 No. 1523 and 1977 Nos. 675, 1039 and 1053.

Manufacturer's licence

Section 19 requires that in considering an application for a manufacturer's licence the licensing authority must have regard to the premises and equipment of the manufacturer, to the qualifications of his supervisory staff, and the safe-keeping and storage of medicinal products. A licence is required by anyone manufacturing or assembling a medicinal product and that person must also hold a product licence for the particular product or be working to the order and specification of the product licence holder. It should be noted that manufacturing does *not* include dissolving or dispensing the product or mixing it with a vehicle for administration. It should also be noted that the licence covers manufacture of the medicinal product itself and no licence is required to prepare the bulk drug or other chemicals used in its manufacture.

The form and contents of an application for a manufacturing licence are laid out in SIs 1971 No. 974 and 1977 No. 1052 and details of the manufacture or assembly procedure must be given, together with the qualifications of the production manager and the person in charge of quality control.

Wholesale dealer's licences

A wholesaler's licence is required by anyone who as a business sells medicinal products by way of wholesale dealing, ie with the intention that they are to be sold again or administered to human beings by way of business. Section 131 provides that the provision of services under the NHS is to be treated as carrying on a business by the Minister, so that supplying the NHS is wholesale dealing. However, a manufacturer does not need a wholesale licence to sell his products, nor does a product licence holder who does not manufacture his own products.

In considering the application for a wholesale dealer's licence Section 19 requires the licensing authority to consider the premises, equipment and storage facilities of the applicant. The application must be made in the form laid out in SIs 1971 No. 974 and 1977 No. 1052.

Clinical trials
Section 31 of the Act defines a clinical trial as an investigation wherein a doctor(s) or dentist(s) administers a medicinal product to one or more patients where there is evidence that the medicinal product may be beneficial and the trial is to determine to what extent it is indeed beneficial and what other effects it may have. The section provides that no-one in the course of a business may sell or supply, procure the sale or supply, or manufacture or procure the manufacture of any medicinal product for the purpose of a clinical trial unless he holds a product licence that authorises the trial or a *clinical trial certificate* has been issued by the licensing authority permitting the trial. Because a clinical trial done under a product licence will be limited to the approved indications and therapeutic uses in that licence, and most clinical trials are to evaluate new indications or uses, a clinical trial certificate is the usual way of permitting a trial. Similarly, a medicinal product may only be imported for use in a clinical trial by someone holding a product licence or a clinical trial certificate authorising the trial.

Section 31 provides that a clinical trial certificate is not required by a doctor or dentist conducting a clinical trial in his own right and not acting at the request of a third party and to this extent a pharmacist at a registered pharmacy (see page 72), hospital or health centre may dispense a doctor's prescription. Similarly, a clinical trial certificate is not required by a manufacturer who prepares a medicinal product for a doctor or dentist or a pharmacist supplying that doctor or dentist acting under this exception. If a practitioner has any doubt he may notify the Medicines Division of his intention (SI 1972 No. 1200).

The contents and form of an application for a clinical trial certificate are given in SIs 1971 No. 973, 1972 No. 1201, 1975 No. 681 and 1977 No. 1051. The application should include detailed information on the chemistry and pharmacy of the substance and details of animal pharmacological and toxicological tests supporting the relative safety of the agent and should show a reason to test it in the human. Details of the proposed clinical trials must also be given.

Fees
All types of licence and certificate are subject to payment of a set of prescribed fees.

Chapter Seven

MEDICINES ACT 1968 (CONTINUED)

Controls on Medicinal Products

Controls on Retail Sales

It was seen in the last chapter that the licensing system only controls sales by manufacturers and by wholesalers. Part III (Ss 51-68) of the Medicines Act which was introduced on 1st February 1978 seeks to control the retail sale and supply of medicinal products. Section 131 defines retail sale and supply as any sale or supply other than for the purpose of resale or resupply or for administration to human beings in the course of a business. Because S131(5) defines the provision of the Health Services as carrying on a business by the Ministers for this purpose, sales to the NHS are not retail sales.

The broad effect of Part III is to require all retail sales of medicinal products to be made from registered pharmacies, but those on the general sales list are exempt this requirement while others may only be supplied on a practitioner's prescription – 'prescription only products'. Before the introduction of Part III the Minister had imposed limitations on the retail sale of certain medicinal products by prohibition orders under the power given him by S62 of the Act. In this way controls had been imposed on both phenacetin and hexachlorophane by SIs 1973 No. 1120, 1974 Nos. 711, 1082 and 2167. These products are now controlled by Part III regulations and the relevant prohibition orders have been repealed. Similarly, together with the introduction of Part III there was the repeal of the Pharmacy and Poisons Act 1933, the Pharmacy and Medicines Act 1941 and the Therapeutic Substances Act 1956, and the introduction of the Poisons Act 1972.

Part III covers human and animal medicines and medicated animal feedstuffs. Only its application to human medicine will be considered here.

Sale and supply of medicinal products

Section 52 provides that no-one may sell, or offer to sell, by retail any medicinal product that is not on the general sales list unless he is lawfully conducting a retail pharmacy business, the sale is made at a registered pharmacy and is made by, or under the supervision, of a pharmacist.

Section 51 permits the appropriate Minister to specify by order which medicinal products are to be on the general sales list and such products must be capable of being sold reasonably safely other than by a pharmacist. The same section also permits the Minister to specify what medicinal products may be sold by means of automatic machines. When general sales list products are sold other than at a registered pharmacy Section 53 requires the place of sale to be the premises where the business is carried on and they must be capable of excluding the public (ie a shop rather than a market stall). Such medicinal products must have been made up elsewhere than at these premises and the contents must not have been opened since made up. Section 54 requires that no-one may offer for sale any medicinal product from an automatic machine unless it is in the automatic machine section of the general sales list.

Exceptions

(i) *Practitioners*
Section 55 provides certain general exceptions to the general sales list and pharmacy-only requirements of Sections 52 and 53. Thus the restrictions on sale or supply or the offer thereof do not apply to doctors or dentists in respect of patients of theirs. Nor do they apply to hospitals or health centres provided supplies are in accordance with the directions of a doctor or dentist. Further, the Ministers may specify certain groups of medicinal products to which the restrictions on sale and supply (but not the offer thereof) do not apply to a registered nurse or a certified midwife (see page 65).

(ii) *Herbal remedies*
Section 56 exempts from the provisions of Sections 52 and 53 the retail sale of herbal remedies from herbalists' shops. The section also empowers the Minister to designate certain herbal remedies to be outside this exemption and SI 1977 No. 2130 lists those substances to which the S56 exemption does not apply.

Other Ministerial powers
Section 60 empowers a Minister to restrict the retail sale and supply of medicinal products of a certain type to specially certified practitioners or someone acting on his instructions who is conducting a retail pharmacy business. This provision is to be used where the sale or supply of a medicinal product requires specialised knowledge on the part of the practitioner and the Minister may specify what qualifications and experience a practitioner should have.

Section 61 empowers a Minister to limit the availability of a class of medicinal products to a certain class of persons.

Section 62 empowers a Minister to issue an order prohibiting the sale, supply or importation of a specified medicinal product. Such a prohibition may be total or subject to such exceptions as the order specifies. The Minister must consult with the appropriate Section 4 committee or the Medicines Commission before making the order or, where it is urgent, may make an immediate order that will have effect for three months. As mentioned above phenacetin and hexachloraphane were the subject of prohibition orders which limited their availability and were replaced by the Part III controls. An example of a permanent prohibition is given by SI 1976 No. 1861 and 1977 No. 670 and concerns the unapproved substance, Bal Jivan Chamcho.

Section 66 gives the Ministers wide powers to regulate such matters as the supervision of dispensing medicinal products, the premises at which they are stored, their safekeeping and disposal, precautions in handling them, the keeping of records of sales and supply, etc.

Sections 67 and 68 make contravention of the provisions of Part III, and regulations made under its powers, an offence, and specify penalties.

Part III Regulations

(i) *Pharmacy only products*
As has already been seen the effect of S52 is to make all medicinal products that are not on the general sales list 'pharmacy only' products, ie they may only be sold or supplied retail by someone conducting a retail pharmacy business when the product must be sold from registered pharmacy (see page 72) by, or under the supervision of, a pharmacist.

(ii) *General Sales List*
The Medicines (General Sales List) Order 1977 SI No. 2129 (as amended by SI 1979 No. 315) contains a list of all those medicinal products that may be sold other than from a retail pharmacy so long as the provisions of S53 (above page 63) are fulfilled. Schedule 1 to the Order includes a variety of proprietary medicines that are on the list, and states where appropriate the maximum number of unit doses (tablets, for example) in each pack. Thus aspirin 300mg tablets must not be sold in packs of more than 25 tablets to be on the general sales list. Schedule 3 consists of five columns: column 1 listing the medicinal products concerned, column 2 the maximum strength permitted as a general sales list product, column 3 the permitted uses or pharmaceutical forms, column 4 the maximum dose and maximum daily dose to be stated, and column 5 the

maximum number of specified dose units to be in a pack. Thus to be on the general sales list paracetamol, for example, for adult use must be in tablet form and must not be sold in packs of more than 25 tablets and each tablet must not contain more than 500mg of the product. If these stipulations are not fulfilled the product must be regarded as a pharmacy-only one. Schedule 5 permits only 'Aspro' and 'Rennies' to be sold from automatic machines.

(iii) *Prescription-only list*

The Medicines (Prescription Only) Order 1977 SI No. 2127 (as amended by SI 1978 No. 189, No. 987 and SI 1979 No. 36) lists those medicinal products that are to be available only on a practitioner's prescription. A practitioner means a doctor, dentist or veterinarian. Schedule 1 to the Order lists the prescription-only products but also indicates the circumstances in which the listed medicinal products may be exempt from this class. These exemptions may be related to the maximum strength, its use or pharmaceutical form and maximum dose or daily dose. Thus the substance, naphazoline hydrochloride, which is prescription-only, is exempted from this restriction when presented as nasal spray or drops not containing liquid paraffin and not in a greater strength than 0.05%. Part II of Schedule 1 lists prescription-only products that are also controlled by the Misuse of Drugs Act 1971 (see chapters 2 and 3). Generally speaking, except for insulin all human medicinal products for injection are prescription-only. The Order makes provision for a pharmacist to supply prescription-only medicines in an emergency without a prescription. Subject to certain conditions the pharmacist may provide three days' supply and the doctor must undertake to provide a proper prescription within 72 hours. An emergency supply cannot be followed by another. The Order also requires a prescription be written in indelible ink and contain the address and signature of the practitioner, be dated, indicate whether the prescriber is a doctor, dentist or veterinarian, give the patient's name and address (and age if under 12). Except for a repeat prescription a prescription must be dispensed within six months of its date.

(iv) *Exceptions*

There is a variety of exceptions to the controls on retail sales and supply outlined above which are given either in the Medicines (Prescription Only) Order 1977 SI No. 2127 or the Medicines (Pharmacy and General Sales List Exemptions) Order 1977 SI No. 2133. The exception for practitioners in S55 has already been noted (page63). The others of importance to the Health Service relate to:

Midwives – Midwives may sell or supply in the course of their profession a variety of specified prescription-only products, mainly the choral-type hypnotics, ergometrine (but not for injection) and the pain killer, pentazocine. In addition she may sell or supply any general sales list or pharmacy-only product.

Hospitals – Prescription medicines may be sold or supplied by a hospital provided they are in accordance with the written instructions of a doctor although these instructions need not be contained in a formal prescription as described above.

Registered ophthalmic opticians – Opticians may sell or supply certain specified prescription-only products in the course of their profession. The products are mainly a series of eye drops and ointments.

Pharmacists – Pharmacists may supply registered ophthalmic opticians with the listed products mentioned above without a prescription, but a signed order is required.

Chiropodists – State registered chiropodists may sell or supply certain general sales and pharmacy-only products listed in the Exemptions Order in the course of their practice.

Other exceptions – Exceptions are made for the sale of medicinal products in high dilution (ie for homeopathic medicine) provided they are not used parenterally. Provision is made for the sale and supply of all medicinal products to universities, research and higher educational institutions, public analysts, sampling officers, medicines inspectors etc. Supply (but not sale) of medicinal products by the masters of ships with no doctors, the lifeboat service and the voluntary ambulance services (for example, St Johns Ambulance and the Red Cross) is also provided for by the Order, subject to certain restrictions.

Other Controls on Medicinal Products

Clearly the safety of a medicinal product can depend upon how it is used and thus the Act seeks to control both sales promotion (Part VI) and labelling, packing and identification of medicinal products (Part V).

Sales Promotion (Part VI – Ss 92-97)

The Act does not define 'promotion' but makes it clear that the term includes both advertisements and representations which are defined by Section 92. 'Advertisement' covers every form of advertising, whether by publication, display of a notice or a catalogue, price list or other document, words or an article or by a photograph, cinema film, sound recording or radio or television broadcast. Advertisement does not include the spoken word except as the sound track of a film or as a broadcast on radio or television. However, representation means any statement or undertaking given by the spoken word except a film soundtrack or a broadcast.

(i) *Offences related to promotion*
Section 94 provides that the only commercially interested party who may advertise, or cause to be advertised, a medicinal product is the product licence holder. Contravention of this requirement is an offence, summary conviction carrying a fine of up to £100.

Section 93 makes it an offence to issue a false or misleading advertisement or representation, or to make an unauthorised recommendation for a medicinal product. A recommendation is unauthorised if it is not permitted by the product licence. On summary conviction there can be a fine of up to £400 and on indictment two years' imprisonment or any fine or both. The section also provides for certain defences to these offences.

(ii) *Ministers' powers to control promotion*
Section 95 of the Act gives the appropriate Minister extensive powers to regulate advertisements and representations concerning medicinal products. Thus he is able to prohibit all advertising of any specified medicinal product or group of them, advertising of medicinal products for certain diseases or the use of certain words or phrases in advertisements. Similarly, representations may be prohibited. The Ministers also have powers to regulate by Order the contents of advertisements, their form and, if they are film or television advertisements, their duration. Contravention of such regulations is an offence liable on summary conviction to a fine of up to £400, or on indictment a term of imprisonment up to two years, any fine or both. Regulations may modify these penalties. The use of these powers is illustrated by the controls on advertising to the public (see below). In order to police this system Section 97 empowers the licensing authority to demand up to 12 copies of any advertisement issued in the previous 12 months, Failure to do so on demand is an offence liable on summary conviction to a fine not exceeding £50.

(iii) *Advertising to the general public*
Promotion of medicinal products to the public is controlled by the Medicines (Labelling and Advertising to the Public) Regulations SI 1978 No. 41. The regulations prohibit advertising to the public of any prescription-only product. They prohibit advertising for the treatment of venereal disease, tuberculosis,

cancer, diabetes, epilepsy or fits, kidney disease, paralysis, cataract or glaucoma. They prohibit advertisements for medicinal products for the treatment of a variety of other conditions, but also specify exceptions. For example, while advertisements for the treatment of diseases of the nervous system are prohibited, advertisements for the symptomatic relief of headache including migraine, are permitted. The regulations also prohibit the use of certain words in advertisements to the public while also requiring certain words or phrases to be used in certain instances. Thus an advertisement may not refer to the Medicines Commission or a Section 4 Committee but in the case of a herbal remedy it must be clearly stated, 'A herbal remedy for . . . '

(iv) *Advertising to doctors*
Section 96 requires that no advertisement shall be sent or representation made to a practitioner by a commercially interested party unless a data sheet relating to the particular medicinal product has been sent or given to the practitioner in the last 15 months, and the advertisement must not be inconsistent with the data sheet. A compendium of data sheets is sent to all doctors annually by the Association of the British Pharmaceutical Industry, and this serves this purpose. A data sheet is a document that the product licence holder is required to prepare which in a standardised format gives certain basic technical data about the product. The form and contents of data sheets are defined in SI 1972 No. 2076. The aim of this requirement is to ensure that before receiving any advertising matter on a product a doctor is in possession of technical information about the product which has been approved by the product licence, and therefore the licensing authority.

The form and content of advertising to doctors is controlled partially by Order (SI 1978 No. 1020) and partially by a strict code of practice. The code of practice is agreed between the DHSS and the Association of the British Pharmaceutical Industry and covers all aspects of promotion of medicinal products to doctors. It should also be noted that advertising may, to some extent, be controlled by the licensing system by introducing standard or other provisions into product licences.

Controls on labelling, containers, etc. Part V (Ss 85-91)

(i) *Labelling*
Section 85 empowers the appropriate Minister to make regulations to control labelling of containers or packages of medicinal products or require distinctive marks to be displayed on them. Such regulations are to be made in order to ensure the medicinal products are correctly described, that any appropriate

warnings are given, that no information is false or misleading and that the safe use of the product is promoted. The section makes it an offence to sell or supply, or to possess for sale or supply, any medicinal product which contravenes these regulations.

Labelling regulations have been made under SIs 1976 No. 1726 and 1977 No. 996, 2168; 1978 No. 41 and 190 and provide for the general form and content of labels for medicinal products and special requirements for medicinal products used for clinical trials.

(ii) *Leaflets*

Section 86 empowers the appropriate Ministers to make regulations controlling the form and content of any leaflets that may be supplied with medicinal products. The section makes it an offence to contravene any such regulations and also to issue a leaflet which falsely describes the product or is likely to mislead.

(iii) *Containers*

Section 87 permits the appropriate Minister to make regulations to prohibit the sale or supply of medicinal products except in containers specified therein. Such regulations are to be designed to ensure that medicinal products are correctly identified and safe. It is an offence to contravene any regulations.

Several Orders have been made under this provision. Statutory Instrument 1975 No. 2000 requires all aspirin and paracetamol preparations for children to be dispensed in standard child-proof containers while SI 1976 No. 1643 extends this requirement to adult aspirin and paracetamol. However, there are certain exceptions for non-retail sale and supply. Statutory Instrument 1978 No. 40 requires that a variety of medicinal products that are liquids for external use must be supplied in fluted bottles. In effect this transfers an earlier requirement of the Pharmacy and Poisons Act 1933 on medicinal poisons to the Medicines Act.

(iv) *Other powers*

A variety of other powers are conferred on the appropriate Minister by Part V. Thus S88 empowers him to make regulations concerning the colour and shape of medicinal products or distinctive marks to be displayed on them while S89 gives him the power to control information exposed on the outside of automatic vending machines. It is an offence to contravene these regulations.

(v) *Penalties*
Section 91 provides that offences against Sections 85 or 86, or any regulation made under Sections 85, 86 or 87 on summary conviction, are liable to a fine not exceeding £400. On indictment a term of imprisonment of up to two years, any fine or both are possible. Regulations may specify lesser penalties.

Liability For Harm Caused By Medicinal Products

Although the Medicines Act is designed to increase among other things the level of safety associated with medicinal products, and to this end creates a variety of criminal offences, it does not affect the civil liability arising from harm caused by medicines. The law of negligence deals with the extent to which a manufacturer, prescriber or hospital may be liable for any harm caused by a medicinal product.

Donoghue v Stevenson 1932

In the important case of *Donoghue v Stevenson 1932* a bottle of ginger beer had been sold by the defendant to someone who gave it to the plaintiff. The plaintiff, after drinking some and then pouring it out, found it contained a decomposed snail and suffered shock and gastroenteritis. The question was to what extent was the manufacturer liable in the law of tort. On appeal to the House of Lords Lord Atkin held that there was a general duty on everyone to take reasonable care to avoid acts or omissions which might reasonably be foreseen as likely to cause injury to his neighbour. In law he held that a neighbour was anyone so closely and directly connected with a person's actions or omissions that that person should reasonably take him into consideration when considering their consequences. The court found that a manufacturer of products intended to reach the consumer in the form in which they left him with no reasonable possibility of intermediate examination owes a duty to the consumer to take reasonable care.

This is the position of any manufacturer including one of pharmaceutical products. If he has taken reasonable care to ensure his product will not harm the consumer he will not be liable for any damage that actually occurs. What is reasonable care is a matter of fact in each case, but generally it requires him to take all reasonable steps that any careful and skilful manufacturer would take to avoid foreseeable damage.

Congenital Disabilities (Civil Liability) Act 1976

The thalidomide case in which unborn children were injured by the drug raised another issue: Does a defendant owe a duty of care to an unborn child? In 1972 both Canadian (*Duval v Seguin*) and Australian (*Watt v Rama*) cases decided that such a duty was owed, but no English court has ever decided on the point. Thus the thalidomide case was settled out of court, and in the recent case of *Williams v Luff (TLR 14 Feb. 1978)* where the pre-natal injury arose from a car accident, the defendant admitted liability, avoiding the need for a judicial ruling on the question. However, the Congenital Disabilities (Civil Liability) Act 1976 has provided by statute that a duty of care is owed to the unborn child.

Negligence in Prescribing

The position of a doctor or other person prescribing a medicinal product is also covered by the law of negligence. In such a case the prescriber owes a duty to the patient to take such care and use such skill as any careful prescriber would adopt in the particular circumstances. What is reasonable care and skill would depend on the precise facts of the situation, but a greater degree of care would be required for a new and only partially proven drug, or one with a known danger, than for one that was well established and relatively innocuous.

Moves Towards "Strict Liability"

There is presently a general move towards the imposition of strict liability in place of the tort of negligence in this area. Thus an EEC directive proposes that a producer of a defective product should be liable for the damage his product causes, irrespective of whether he has been negligent or not. The Law Commission and the Scottish Law Commission (Law Com. No. 82, and Scot. Law Com. No. 45) have considered this Directive and, while finding difficulties with the EEC proposals, have made the point that no difference should be drawn between pharmaceutical and other products. Similarly, the Royal Commission on Civil Liability and Personal Injury under Lord Pearson have recommended an extension of the principle of no fault liability. This may well, therefore, be the pattern for the future.

Other Provisions of the Medicines Act

Retail pharmacy

We have already seen that Part III of the Medicines Act deals with the retail sale and supply of medicinal products and that generally such sales are limited to persons lawfully conducting a retail pharmacy business, the sale being made from a registered pharmacy by or under the supervision of, a pharmacist. A pharmacist is defined by section 132 as someone on the register of pharmaceutical chemists established by the Pharmacy Act 1852 and maintained by the Pharmacy Act 1954 which regulates the profession of pharmacy. Part IV of the Medicines Act (Ss 69-84) deals with the definition of a lawful retail pharmacy business, of a registered pharmacy and a variety of incidental matters.

(i) *Retail Pharmacy Business*
Section 132 defines a retail pharmacy business as one which consists of, or includes, the retail sale of medicinal products other than those on a general sales list. If general sales list products are also sold the business is still a retail pharmacy. However, a professional practice carried on by a practitioner who supplies medicinal products (a dispensing doctor, for example) is not a retail pharmacy business. Section 69 provides that such a business may be lawfully carried on by a pharmacist, a partnership of pharmacists, a corporate body (provided the dispensing of medicinal products is under the management of a superintendent pharmacist) or the personal representative of a deceased, bankrupt or mentally ill pharmacist. Thus, except for the last case, a retail pharmacy business must be carried on by a pharmacist, and Section 70 requires that sales of medicinal products (except general sales list products) must be under the personal control of a pharmacist and that his name and certificate of registration (under the Pharmacy Act 1954) be conspicuously exhibited. Section 71 requires the same in the case of a corporate body for the superintendent pharmacist. In the case of a business being carried on by the personal representatives of a pharmacist, Section 72 requires that the sale and supply of medicinal products (except general sales list products) be under the personal control of a pharmacist whose name and certificate is also prominently displayed.

Provided the owner of a retail pharmacy business complies with the above conditions he is considered to be lawfully conducting it for the purposes of the Medicines Act.

(ii) *Registration of premises*
We have already seen that a retail pharmacy business must be carried out from registered premises. Sections 74 and 75 deal with the registration of premises and impose a duty on the Registrar of the Pharmaceutical Society of Great Britain to keep a register. Application for registration of a pharmacy must be made in the form prescribed by Orders and must include details of the name and address of the person intending to carry on the business, the name of the pharmacist(s) under whose supervision the business is to be carried on, the address of the premises, the date of intended commencement of business and a description of the premises including a sketch map showing the areas where medicinal products are to be sold, supplied, prepared, dispensed and stored. The registrar notifies the Minister, and no entry may be made in the register for two

months, and not at all unless the registrar is reasonably satisfied that the applicant is, or will be, lawfully conducting a retail pharmacy business. If the Minister believes that the premises do not fulfil the regulations made under S66 concerning the standards of retail pharmacy premises he must within the two-month period give notice to the applicant that he proposes to certify that the premises are unfit. The applicant has 28 days in which to lodge an appeal.

A retention fee is payable in respect of premises and Sections 80-83 deal with the disqualification of premises and removals from the register.

(iii) *Titles etc.*
Part IV also deals with the use of certain descriptions or titles in Section 78. The word 'pharmacy' may be used only in respect of a registered pharmacy or the pharmaceutical department of a hospital or health centre. Only a pharmacist may use the titles 'pharmaceutical chemist', 'pharmaceutist', 'pharmacist' or 'Member or Fellow of the Pharmaceutical Society'. The title, 'chemist and druggist', 'druggist', 'dispensing chemist' or 'dispensing druggist', may be used only by someone conducting a retail pharmacy business. Powers are given to the Health Ministers to increase or relax these restrictions after consultation with the Pharmaceutical Society.

The British Pharmacopoeia
The British Pharmacopoeia (the BP) is an alphabetical collection of monographs on certain commonly used medicinal products each of which sets certain technical standards for these products. Formerly the BP was compiled by the General Medical Council (the GMC) under the provisions of Section 47 of the Medical Act 1956. Section 98 of the Medicines Act 1968 transfers the copyright in the BP from the GMC to Her Majesty. Section 99 provides that new editions are to be prepared by the 'appropriate body' which is a Section 4 body, the British Pharmacopoeia Commission (SI 1970 No. 1256). As has already been seen (see page 54) the Commission has a large number of specialist committees working on the publication.

Section 101 provides that the Medicines Commission or a Section 4 committee acting under the direction of the Medicines Commission may prepare any other publications relevant to medicinal products and the Minister may cause it to be made available for sale to the public or otherwise distribute it.

Radioactive Substances and the Medicines Act

The Radioactive Substances Act 1948 prohibits the administration of any radioactive substance by way of treatment unless it is done by a licensed practitioner or someone acting under his direction (S3). Similarly S4 limits the use of irradiating apparatus to licensed practitioners. Statutory Instruments 1978 Nos. 1004, 1005 and 1006 bring the control of radioactive medicinal products under the Medicines Act and sets up a new Section 4 Committee on radiation.

Radioactive Substances

Section 104(1) of the Medicines Act permits the Ministers by regulation to extend the provisions of the Act to substances that while not medicinal products as defined by S130(1) are partly or wholly used for a medicinal purpose. The Medicines (Radioactive Substances) Order 1978 (SI 1978 No. 1004) uses this power to extend the application of S60 of the Act (which limits the sale, supply and administration of substances specified by order to practitioners holding a certificate issued by the appropriate Minister) to certain substances or articles consisting of or containing radioactive substances. These are listed in the Schedule to the order, and include radioactive substances in containers for internal or surface application and apparatus designed to generate neutrons for diagnostic or research purposes. The order modifies the definition of 'administer' given in S130(9) of the Act to include exposure of the body or any part thereof to neutrons emitted by the apparatus.

Control of Administration

The Medicines (Administration of Radioactive Substances) Regulation 1978 (SI 1978 No. 1006) made under the power contained in S60 of the Medicines Act controls the administration of radioactive medicinal products. Regulation 2 (from 1.7.80) provides that no person shall administer to a human being (other than himself) any radioactive medicinal product unless he is a doctor or dentist holding a certificate issued by the Health Ministers or is a person acting in accordance with the direction of such a person. Holders of certificates may only administer such radioactive medicinal products, for such purposes as are specified in the certificate.

Issue of Certificates

Regulation 4 (effective from 1.7.80) lays down the procedure for the issue of certificates. Application must be in writing signed by the applicant and in the approved form. The applicants name and address, qualifications, experience and the position he holds must be stated. The classes of radioactive medicinal products he proposes to administer and for what purpose, and details of the equipment, staff and facilities available to him must be specified. If the Health Ministers are satisfied he is fit to hold a licence, that he has suitable facilities available to him, and are satisfied with the radiation hazard then they may grant the certificate. They may specify in the certificate the types of radioactive medicinal product or the purposes of administration to which it applies.

Regulation 5 deals with the duration and renewal of certificates. Certificates normally remain in force for 5 years and may be renewed on written application provided there have been no changes in the particulars specified in the original application.

Regulation 6 provides that the Health Ministers may suspend or revoke a certificate where a material change has occurred in a matter stated in the application or the holder no longer has suitable facilities or staff available to him. The Minister also has the power to vary a certificate.

Regulation 7 provides that where the Health Ministers refuse to grant or renew a certificate or suspend, vary or revoke one the applicant or holder may appeal in person or writing against the decision to a person appointed for the purpose.

Advisory Committee

In order to advise the Health Ministers on matters relating to the issue of certificates regulation 3 sets up the Administration of Radioactive Substances Advisory Committee. The majority of the Committee are to be doctors and must include persons with wide and recent experience of radioactive substances. The chairman of the committee is to be a doctor.

The Committee on Radiation from Radioactive Medicinal Products

Under the power in S4(1) of the Medicines Act, the Medicines (Committee on Radiation from Radioactive Medicinal Products) Order 1978 (SI 1978 No. 1005) establishes this Committee. The function of the CRRMP is to give advice on the safety, quality and efficacy, in relation to radiation, of any substance or article for human use to which any provision of the Medicines Act is applicable.

Chapter Eight

Controls on Alcohol:

METHYLATED SPIRITS AND INTOXICATING LIQUORS

Introduction

Unlike dangerous drugs, poisons and medicinal products whose control is fairly recent, alcohol has been subject to controls for many hundreds of years. However, it was not (and still is not) the undoubted abuse potential of this substance that led to its control but its potential to raise revenue for the Exchequer in the form of excise duty.

Alcohol, particularly in the form of sherry wine, was once widely used in pharmacy as a vehicle for medicines. It is rarely used in this way today now that solid preparations of medicines, such as tablets and capsules, have taken over from liquids. However, alcohol in the form of methylated spirits is still widely used in medicine both to sterilise and harden the skin, and also as an ingredient in a variety of external preparations. In addition, pure alcohol (ethyl alcohol or ethanol) is widely used in hospital laboratories and in the preparation of some medicines.

In this chapter a broad summary of the controls imposed on alcohol in its various forms will be given. The main Acts concerned were the Customs and Excise Act 1952 and the Licensing Act 1953 and Regulations made under both, but recently the law on alcohol has been consolidated in the Alcoholic Liquor Duties Act 1979.

Controls on Methylated Spirits

Definitions and general aspects

Methylated spirits are spirits (i.e. alcohol prepared by distillation) that have been denatured by the addition of various noxious substances to make them unsuitable for consumption. They are intended for industrial, medical and household use, and because they cannot be used for drinking they may be exempted from the excise duty on spirits imposed by section 5 of the Alcoholic Liquor Duties Act (see S9).

Methylated spirits may be manufactured or sold wholesale only by someone holding a licence issued by the Commissioners of Customs and Excise (S75). Moreover, S76 provides that no person may sell by retail methylated spirits unless he holds a licence. The Act gives the local Customs and Excise officer powers to enter and inspect premises of any holder of a licence. He may examine stocks and records and take samples (for which he must pay). The regulations provide for the safekeeping and control of methylated spirits on retailers' premises, and also for a system of disposal in the event of closure of the business or death of the proprietor.

Section 79 of the Alcoholic Liquor Duties Act makes it unlawful to deal with methylated spirits in any of the following ways:

(i) to prepare or sell any methylated spirits for use as a beverage or mixed with a beverage;

(ii) to use methylated spirits to prepare any article capable of being used as a beverage or as a medicine for internal use, or to sell or possess any such article;

(iii) to purify, or attempt to purify, methylated spirits, or attempt to receive the alcohol in it by distillation, condensation or any other means.

Some five types of methylated spirits are defined by the regulations but we need deal with only two here. On the one hand there is mineralised methylated spirits which is the only type available to the public. On the other there is industrial methylated spirits which is not available to the general public but is the type used in pharmacy for a variety of topical preparations.

Industrial methylated spirits (IMS)

Industrial methylated spirits (IMS) consists of 95 parts by volume of spirits and 5 parts wood naphtha to denature it. In the pure 'Q' grade of IMS 5% methyl alcohol replaces the naphtha. A bitter tasting agent, quassin, is added to make IMS unpalatable. Wood naphtha and methyl alcohol are poisonous. IMS is not available on retail sale to the public and virtually all dealings with IMS have to be authorised by the Commissioners of Customs and Excise.

Retail pharmacy business

A retail pharmacy business may only receive IMS if authorised to do so by the Commissioners of Custom and Excise. It must be purchased from either an authorised methylator (ie the manufacturer) in quantities not less than five gallons and not more than 200 gallons at a time, or from an authorised wholesaler in quantities of not more than four gallons at a time. Orders must be on a special requisition supplied by the Customs and Excise officer. Having been authorised to receive IMS a retail pharmacy may then deal with it in the following ways:

Sale. A retail pharmacy may sell up to four gallons of IMS to a person authorised by the Commissioners to receive it. A requisition must be tendered and retained and the container must be labelled 'industrial methylated spirits'. Up to half a gallon may also be sold to a doctor, dentist or veterinarian, or hospital or nursing home on presentation of an order signed by a practitioner. Such an order must not be more than one week old and only one quantity may be supplied per order.

Dispensing. A retail pharmacist will need a further authority to prepare articles containing IMS, or to dispense IMS or articles containing it. Such products can be supplied only on a practitioner's prescription unless they are 'approved' products (see later).

Sale and supply on prescription. An authorised retail pharmacist may sell or supply either preparations containing IMS or IMS itself (whether diluted or not) to a prescription of a doctor, dentist or veterinarian. The prescription must be signed and dated. If the prescription is for a preparation containing IMS not more than one pint as ingredient may be supplied. If it is not an NHS prescription the name of the patient, the name of the prescriber and the date must be entered in the prescription book. The product must be labelled 'for external use only' or 'not to be taken'. If the prescription is for IMS itself the quantity to be supplied must be stated and in any case not more than one pint may be supplied. The prescription should not be more than one week old and, if not an NHS prescription, it must be kept for two years. The container must be labelled 'for external use only'.

Sale and supply of approved articles. Provided a retail pharmacist is authorised to do so by the Commissioners he may prepare and sell certain products containing IMS that are approved by regulations. The best known of these products is probably surgical spirits (which while freely available in England is limited in Scotland–see later) but it also includes a variety of lotions, liniments, paints, varnishes and analytical chemical reagents. There are special labelling requirements for the various categories of approved product including the need to label them either 'for external use only' or 'not to be taken'.

Practitioners and hospitals

As has already been seen, a doctor, dentist, veterinarian, hospital or nursing home may obtain up to half a gallon of IMS from a retail or wholesale chemist on presentation of an order signed by a practitioner.

Any practitioner, hospital or nursing home may apply to the Customs and Excise office to be authorised to receive IMS for making up articles to be dispensed for medical, surgical, dental or veterinary use other than for administration internally as a medicine. If this authority has been obtained then supplies of between five and 200 gallons may be obtained directly from a methylator as in the case of a retail pharmacist. The same conditions that apply to dispensing IMS and IMS-containing products by a retailer apply to an authorised practitioner or hospital.

Mineralised methylated spirits

Mineralised methylated spirits (MMS) is the only type of methylated spirits that can be sold to the public. It is dyed a distinctive colour and given a distinctive odour to make it unpalatable. As with all methylated spirits consumption can lead to blindness. It may be sold retail to the public in England and Wales without any formality by anyone holding a licence issued by the local Customs and Excise office. A licence will not be issued until the local officer is satisfied that the premises of the applicant are suitable for the storage and sale of MMS.

In Scotland, where methylated spirits drinking has always been a problem there are additional restrictions on the sale of MMS, and also on surgical spirit (an 'approved' article containing IMS – see earlier). Sales in Scotland may only lawfully be made by someone conducting a retail pharmacy business or whose name is on a local authority list kept for the purpose. The sale must be made at these premises and a record made of the date of sale, name and address of the purchaser, the quantity supplied and the purpose for which it is required. The purchaser's signature must also be obtained. (Methylated Spirits (Sale by Retail) (Scotland) Act 1937)

Controls on Pure Alcohol

Pure alcohol (ethyl alcohol, ethanol) comes within the legal term 'spirits' and may be required in the health service for use in preparation of a variety of pharmaceutical substances or for use in laboratories. It is possible to purchase ethanol duty-free if the intended use is approved by the Customs and Excise office and authority obtained to receive it. Application must be made on the appropriate form and details of the proposed use, where it is to be stored and the likely annual requirements must be given. The usual conditions imposed by the Customs and Excise office is that it must be kept in a locked area and that access is limited to certain personnel from whom all supplies must be obtained. A stock record sheet showing all quantities obtained and used must be kept. Alternatively, alcohol may have to be bought duty-paid and the duty may be reclaimed in certain circumstances. (Alcoholic Liquors Duties Act Ss 7 and 8)

Controls on Intoxicating Liquors

In effect, intoxicating liquors are controlled in two ways – firstly by artifically inflating the price with either an excise duty (if produced in this country) or a customs duty (if imported), and secondly by means of the licensing laws which seek to limit the availability of intoxicating beverages to the public to certain hours, certain places and people above a certain age. However, as has already been seen, the controls on alcoholic beverages stem less from a desire to limit their potential danger than to collect revenue. The licensing laws are covered in the Licensing Act 1953 while the duty on intoxicating liquors is dealt with in the Alcoholic Liquor Duties Act 1979.

Controls on retail sales

Section 148 of the Customs and Excise Act 1952 provides that no-one may sell intoxicating liquor unless he holds an appropriate excise licence. In England and Wales these are issued by the licensing justices and in Scotland by the licensing court. The licensing authority has an absolute discretion to grant or refuse a licence. If it is intended to sell intoxicating liquors retail an additional retailer's licence is necessary. However, if the proper duty is paid the Commissioners of Customs and Excise must grant a retailer's licence to anyone holding an excise licence.

The retailer's licence will be subject to a variety of conditions and stipulations. It may authorise sales on or off the premises and it may stipulate maximum and minimum quantities to be sold. Sales may be only within the permitted licencing hours; these may vary from place to place and are set by the local licensing justices. The licence holder must display on his premises his name and the nature of his licence.

Exemptions to the retail controls

An excise licence and therefore a retailer's licence is not required for the following:

(i) the sale, wholesale or retail, of perfumes, whatever their alcohol content;

(ii) the sale, wholesale or retail, of alcoholic flavouring essences not intended to be used as, or mixed with, intoxicating liquors;

(iii) the sale, wholesale or retail, of wines or spirits so medicated as to be, in the opinion of the Commissioners, intended for use as medicine and not a beverage. The Commissioners take a strict interpretation of this definition. Of course, a medicated wine or spirit may well be a medicinal product under the Medicines Act and be subject to its provisions;

(iv) the sale of spirits of wine (ethyl alcohol) for medicinal or scientific purposes by persons lawfully conducting a retail pharmacy business. However, the Commissioners may impose conditions on such sales, and in any case not more than 5 ounces may be sold at a time;

(v) the sale by a registered pharmacist or practitioner of medicated or methylated spirits or spirits made up into a medicine;

(vi) the sale of liquors that have been so treated that they can no longer be regarded as an intoxicating liquor.

Exemption from spirits duty

It has already been noted that either customs or excise duty is payable on spirits, but that those used in the production of methylated spirits and methylated spirits itself are exempt. Also in some cases pure alcohol may be bought duty-free (see page 79). The duty is paid by the licensed distiller. If anyone can prove to the satisfaction of the Commissioners that he has used spirits on which duty has been paid to prepare an article for use for medical purposes or used the spirits for a scientific purpose then he may reclaim part or all of the duty. What are recognised medical articles or recognised scientific purposes can only be determined in a particular case by reference to the local Customs and Excise office. (Alcoholic Liquor Duties Act 1979 S8).

Chapter Nine

Miscellaneous Controls

ON POISONS, DRUGS, MEDICINES AND ALCOHOL

Introduction

The Misuse of Drugs Act 1971, the Poisons Act 1972, the Medicines Act 1968, the Licensing Act 1953, the Customs and Excise Act 1952 and the Alcoholic Liquor Duties Act 1979 provide a comprehensive body of legal controls on drugs, poisons, medicinal products and alcohol. However, there are many areas they do not cover. For instance, a person may obtain a substance perfectly legally and then misuse it in some way. The misuse may be as common as being drunk in a public place (contrary to Section 12 of the Licensing Act 1872) or more serious, such as using the substance to procure an illegal abortion or even to kill someone.

To cover these and other various eventualities a body of law has been built up which provides a variety of additional controls on these substances. Some of the more important of these are considered in this chapter.

Administering Poison

The Offences Against the Person Act 1861 creates two separate offences relating to the illegal administration of poison:

a. Section 23 makes it an offence to 'unlawfully administer to, or cause to be administered to or taken by, any other person any poison or other noxious thing so as thereby to endanger the life of such a person, or so as thereby to inflict upon such person grevious bodily harm'. The offence is punishable by up to 10 years' imprisonment.

b. Section 24 makes it an offence to do the same as in Section 23 but 'with intent to injure, aggrieve or annoy such person'. The penalty for this offence is up to five years' imprisonment.

Section 25 of the Act provides that someone charged with an offence under S23 may be convicted under S24 but not vice-versa.

The courts have given particular attention to certain aspects of the definition of these offences:

Poison or other noxious thing. It was held in *R v Cramp 1880* that this phrase included any recognised poison or any substance which is harmful in the quantity administered. In this case it was found that oil of juniper, while not a poison, could be a noxious thing if given in sufficient quantity. If the accused erroneously supposes the substances to be a poison or noxious substance that may amount to an attempt. In *R v Weatherall 1968* a sleeping tablet was held not to be a noxious substance but it would have been otherwise if many such tablets had been given.

Administered. The accused need not administer the substance himself. Thus the offence was committed in both *R v Harley 1830* and *R v Dele 1852* where the substance was left for the victim to take himself. This amounts to 'causing it to be taken'. It would appear from the old case of *Cadman 1825* that a poison intended to be swallowed is not administered until it is taken into the stomach, although this point is uncertain.

With intent to injure, aggrieve etc. It would appear from the case law that this phrase is limited to the physical effects of the substance itself. Thus in *R v Weatherall 1968* the accused put a sleeping tablet in the victim's tea so he could search her handbag for evidence of adultery. When he was charged under Section 23 it was held that this was not with intent to injure, aggrieve or annoy as the tablet did not have this direct physical effect.

Illegal and Legal Abortion

Medicallv an abortion is usually defined as the termination of a pregnancy at any time up to the stage at which the foetus is viable, ie. capable of an independent existence. After this stage the terms, premature birth or premature stillbirth, are used. An abortion or a premature birth may be spontaneous or artifically induced.

The legal definition of abortion is different and covers the termination of pregnancy at any stage from conception to birth by artificial means. There is also an offence of child destruction – Section 1, Infant Life (Preservation) Act 1929 – which deals with the killing of a child capable of being born alive but before it has a separate existence.

It is the offences related to illegal abortion that impinge on the use of poisons and medicines and three such offences are defined in The Offences Against the Person Act 1861:

The offences

(i) Section 58 provides that 'every woman being with child who, with intent to procure her own miscarriage, shall unlawfully administer to herself any poison or other noxious thing, or shall unlawfully use any instrument or other means whatsoever with the like intent . . . shall be guilty of an offence . . . subject to imprisonment for life'.

(ii) Section 58 also provides ' . . . whosoever, with intent to procure the miscarriage of any woman, whether she be or be not with child, shall unlawfully administer to her, or cause to be taken by her, any poison or other noxious thing, or shall unlawfully use any instrument or other means whatsoever with the like intent, shall be guilty of an offence . . . subject to life imprisonment'.

(iii) Section 59 provides that 'whosoever shall unlawfully supply or procure any poison or other noxious thing, or any instrument or other thing whatsoever, knowing that the same is intended to be used unlawfully or employed with intent to procure the miscarriage of any woman, whether she be or be not with child, shall be guilty of an offence subject to imprisonment for 5 years'.

It must be noted that in the first two offences (i and ii) the offence is not one of procuring an abortion but of *administering etc* a substance or *using* an instrument etc with the necessary intent. Certain other points must also be noted:

Pregnant or not. For a woman to commit an offence in respect of herself she must actually be pregnant (with child) but for the other two offences (ii and iii) she need not be so. However, the effect of this distinction was reduced by two court decisions. In *R v Whitchurch 1890* it was held that a non-pregnant woman may be convicted of conspiring with another to procure her own abortion, while in *R v Sockett 1908* it was held that a non-pregnant woman may be convicted of aiding and abetting the offence upon herself by another. Thus, where others are concerned, the woman herself may be liable although not herself pregnant. It does not ever seem to have been decided whether a non-pregnant woman could be convicted of an attempt at the offence on herself where no-one else was involved. However, it should be noted that a woman herself is rarely charged with the offence these days, and in any case conspiracy with a victim was abolished by the Criminal Law Act 1977.

Poison or other noxious thing. The definition of this phrase has been dealt with on Page 83, so that poison means any recognised poison whatever dose is given while 'other noxious thing' means any substance actually harmful at the quantity given. However, it was made clear in *R v Marlow 1964* that the poison or other thing need not be an abortifacient.

Instrument or other means. 'Other means' have been held to include the fingers of the hand in *R v Spicer 1955.* It does not matter that the instrument or other means used were in effect incapable of producing an abortion.

Unlawful: the Abortion Act 1967. All three offences require the said administration or use to be unlawful. Before 1967 any such administration or use coming within the definition of Sections 58 and 59 were unlawful except as defined in the case of *R v Bourne 1939.* In that case a girl had been raped and became pregnant. An eminent doctor had performed an abortion and had been indicted. His successful defence was that it was justifiable in that continuation of the pregnancy would have made the girl a physical and mental wreck and that this threatened her life. Thus, from 1938 to 1967, a defence to a charge associated with abortion was that it was done in good faith for the purpose of preserving the life or health of the woman.

This definition was replaced in 1967 by the provisions of the Abortion Act. Section 1 of that Act provides that no offence under Sections 58 or 59 of the Offences Against the Person Act 1861 is committed 'when a pregnancy is terminated by a registered medical practitioner if two registered medical practitioners both are of the opinion formed in good faith (a) that the continuance of the pregnancy would involve risk to the life of the pregnant woman or of injury to the physical or mental health of the pregnant woman or any existing child of her family greater than if the pregnancy were terminated or (b) that there is a substantial risk that if the child were born it would suffer from such physical or mental abnormality as to be seriously handicapped.' Thus, any act that would otherwise be an offence under Sections 58 and 59 will be lawful if done under the provisions of Section 1 of the Abortion Act.

Knowingly supplying or procuring, S59 It was held in *R v Mills 1963* that to procure a poison etc means to get possession of it. Thus, it does not cover the act of taking an instrument out of a cupboard if it is already in that person's possession.

The requirement that it must be known that it is intended to use the substance or thing unlawfully has been interpreted widely. Thus in *R v Hillman 1863* it was held that it was enough that the accused believed it was for an unlawful purpose although there was evidence that the person supplied did not intend such a use. Similarly, in *R v Titley 1880* it made no difference that the person supplied was a policeman who obtained the thing by false representations about a fictitious woman.

Drugs and Sexual Intercourse

The Sexual Offences Act 1956 deals with a variety of offences, particularly that of rape. However, Section 4(1) provides that 'it is an offence for a person to apply or administer to, or cause to be taken by, a woman any drug, matter or thing with intent to stupefy or overpower her so as thereby to enable any man to have unlawful sexual intercourse with her'.

The offence consists of the *administration etc* with the ulterior intent and it is irrelevant whether sexual intercourse follows or not. It is also clear that the accused need not be the man who intends to have unlawful sexual intercourse, and, of course, the offence may be committed by a woman.

Unlawful sexual intercourse means outside the marriage bond in this context. It will be noted that the phrase 'any drug, matter or thing' is very wide and would certainly include alcohol. There is no requirement that the material should be capable of stupefying etc the woman; only the intent to do so is required.

Drugs Drink and Driving

The adverse effects of alcohol on driving skills is well known, and many drugs and medicines may have the same effect. The Road Traffic Act 1972 is the statute that deals with road traffic offences and it creates three main driving offences – causing death by reckless or dangerous driving (S1), reckless or dangerous driving (S2) and careless and inconsiderate driving (S3). Clearly any of these offences may arise from the consumption of alcohol, drugs or certain medicines. However, the Act specifically creates two driving offences directly related to the consumption of alcohol or drugs – driving under the influence of drink or drugs and driving with a blood alcohol in excess of the prescribed limit. Both of these offences are considered further:

Driving or being in charge when under the influence of drink or drugs
Section 5 of the Road Traffic Act 1972 provides:

S5(1) 'A person who, when driving or attempting to drive a motor vehicle on a road or other public place, is unfit to drive through drink or drugs shall be guilty of an offence';

S5(2) 'Without prejudice to subsection (1) above, a person who, when in charge of a motor vehicle which is on a road or other public place, is unfit to drive through drink or drugs shall be guilty of an offence.'

Unfit to drive is defined by Section 5(4) as meaning that the ability to drive properly is for the time being impaired. The term, drug, was defined in *Armstrong v Clark 1957* as any medicine given to cure, alleviate or assist an ailing body and includes natural substances such as insulin. Thus, a diabetic subject who was unfit due to taking too much insulin would have committed an offence if he drove, attempted to drive or was in charge of a motor vehicle. An interesting case is *Watmore v Jenkins 1962* in which a diabetic had developed infective hepatitis and was taking hydrocortisone which increased his insulin requirements. Evidence was given that while he was driving his liver function improved and his cortisone level fell so that in effect he had too much insulin in his body and became unfit to drive. It was held by the court that his unfitness to drive was not due to drugs (ie his insulin) but to a change in his bodily equilibrium and he was acquitted. However, a diabetic or anyone taking drugs or medicines that are known to impair driving ability should be cautious and ideally should not drive. Any doctor or other medical personnel prescribing such drugs should warn the patient of the dangers. Product licences issued under the Medicines Act 1968 and the labelling regulations require that appropriate warnings are put on drugs that impair driving or other skills (for example, working moving machinery).

Driving or being in charge with an excessive blood alcohol level

Section 6 of the Road Traffic Act 1972 deals solely with alcohol and provides:

S6(1) If a person drives or attempts to drive a motor vehicle on a road or other public place, having consumed alcohol in such a quantity that the proportion thereof in his blood, as ascertained from a laboratory test for which he subsequently provides a specimen under Section 9 of this Act, exceeds the prescribed limit at the time he provided the specimen, he shall be guilty of an offence;

S6(2) without prejudice to subsection (1) above, if a person is in charge of a motor vehicle on a road or other public place having consumed alcohol as aforesaid, he shall be guilty of an offence.

It will be noted that as far as these offences are concerned it is irrelevant whether or not the accused is fit to drive.

Breath tests

Section 8 gives a police constable in uniform a power to administer a breath test if he suspects any person driving or attempting to drive to have alcohol in his body, or suspects him of having committed a traffic offence while the vehicle was in motion. In the latter case the test must be applied as soon as practicable after the commission of the offence. Also, where there has been an accident due to the presence of a motor vehicle on the road or other public place the constable may apply a breath test to anyone he believes was driving or attempting to drive at the time. Where there has been an accident a police constable may administer a breath test to the driver at or near the scene of the accident, at a police station or, if the driver has been taken to hospital, in the hospital. In the latter case the medical officer must be notified and may object to the administration of the test if he thinks it would be prejudicial to the driver's proper care or treatment. If the breath test appears positive the constable may arrest the driver, except where he is a hospital patient.

Blood and urine tests

Section 9 provides that where someone has been arrested under Section 5 or 8 of the Road Traffic Act he may be required by a police constable while at the police station or in a hospital to provide a blood or urine specimen for laboratory test for alcohol, if a previous breath test was positive or he has refused to take such a test. However, where the driver is in hospital the medical officer in charge must be notified and may object on the grounds that such a test may be prejudicial to the person's proper care and treatment. Failure to provide a specimen without reasonble cause is an offence, but the driver must be warned that failure to comply is indeed an offence possibly making him liable to a fine, imprisonment or disqualification. At the present time the prescribed limit of alcohol is 80 milligrammes per one hundred millilitres of blood or, where a urine test is done, the quantity in the urine is converted by standard tables to its equivalent in the blood.

Drink Drugs and Legal Capacity

An individual's mental state at a particular time is often important in law. Probably the two best known examples are the plea of insanity to a criminal offence and the requirement that someone making a will should be of 'sound mind'. However, many other sections of the law are concerned with mental state. Clearly alcohol and drugs and some medicines may lead to alterations in a person's mental state, ranging from reversible intoxication to a permanent mental impairment which may amount to insanity in the eyes of the law.

Some of the commoner examples of how drink, drugs and medicines may affect legal capacity are now considered.

Criminal law

We have already seen that intoxication itself may be a constituent of an offence (for example, drunken driving) and in *DPP v Beard 1920* the court stated that the mere fact that the accused's self-control was diminished by drink was no defence. However, intoxication from any cause may offer a defence in one of two ways, either by negating some necessary mental element of a crime (the mens rea) or by producing insanity within its legal definition.

Mens rea

A crime is made up of two parts – the prohibited act or actus reus, and a necessary accompanying mental element, the guilty mind or the mens rea. Generally speaking, mens rea is made up of one or more of three requirements; the accused must have acted voluntarily, he must have foresight of the consequences of his act, and in some cases he must have a specific ulterior intent. To give an example, burglary involves the entry of a building with the intention of committing theft. The entry must be voluntary, so someone who is unwillingly thrown through a window into a building by someone else hardly enters it voluntarily. Similarly, he must have the ulterior intent to commit theft, and without this it cannot be burglary. Similarly, abortion requires the ulterior intent of causing a miscarriage.

Thus, if intoxication by alcohol, drugs or medicines in some way negates a necessary mental element of a crime it may provide a defence. However, the extent to which this rule is applied would depend upon the particular circumstances of the case. Certainly where the intoxication was deliberately self-induced by the accused to give himself 'Dutch courage' to kill his wife as in *Attorney General for Northern Ireland v Gallagher 1963* this will not be a defence, while at the other extreme, where the intoxication is not self-induced (for example, a drink has been laced, or a medicine given with no appropriate warning) it is very likely to be accepted by the court.

Insanity

The legal definition of insanity is quite unrelated to any medical definition and was first set down in the M'Naghten Rules 1843 – Daniel M'Naghten had shot Sir Robert Peel's secretary in Whitehall in 1843. Because he was insanely deluded he was acquitted and this caused a degree of public disquiet. Because of this, the House of Lords asked the Judges to define the scope of the defence of insanity and this gave rise to the rules. There are three rules: firstly, every man is presumed sane and responsible for his crimes until proved otherwise; secondly, to establish a defence of insanity it must be proved that at the time of the offence the accused was labouring under such a defect of reason from a disease of the mind as not to know the nature and quality of the act he was doing, or if he did know it, that he did not know that what he was doing was wrong; and thirdly, if an accused suffers from insane delusions as to an existing situation then he must be judged as if those delusions were fact.

There has been much legal discussion of these rules by the courts which we cannot deal with here. However, in *DPP v Beard 1920*, which considered drunkenness as a defence, it was held that the law takes no account of the cause of the insanity and it is irrelevent that the accused brought on the insanity himself. It is also clear that insanity within the M'Naghten rules need not be permanent. Thus, where it can be proved that drink or drugs have caused a disease of the mind that has in turn produced a defect of reason such as is described in the rules, then the defence of insanity will be possible. Severe drug addiction, advanced alcoholism or delirium tremens are possible examples.

Tort

Tort is that body of law that is not criminal, whereby rights or duties are imposed upon the public at large that they may enforce against one another by an action in the civil courts. Torts include such things as negligence, defamation and trespass.

No general defence of insanity has been developed in relation to torts and thus the effect of drink or drugs on tortious liability is very limited. Like crimes, torts may have a specific mental element and if drink or drugs negate this they may provide a defence. However, the mental element of most torts is very much less than with most crimes, and in many cases is absent. Thus, the scope of intoxication as a defence here is very limited.

Contract

Generally speaking contract is a sort of private law agreed to between two parties in very specific circumstances but which they may enforce against one another (but no-one else) in a civil court.

The general rule for intoxication is that if at the time of making a contract one party was so intoxicated that he did not know what he was doing, and this was known to the other party, then the contract is voidable. Voidable means that althought the contract is quite legal and valid (unless it suffers from some other defect) it may be repudiated by the party who was intoxicated at the time. However, his right to repudiate will be lost if he confirms the contract in some way as, for example, requiring the other party to perform his part.

Wills

In the case of *Banks v Goodfellow 1870* it was held that for a will to be valid, at the time it is made the testator (ie the person making it) must have a 'sound and disposing mind and memory'. This means that he ought to know the nature of the business he is transacting, what property he has to dispose of and the people he might consider distributing it to. If the effect of drink or drugs is to remove this ability then the will may not be valid. However, it should be noted that a valid will may be made by someone of unsound mind during a lucid period, and someone who has made a will while of unsound mind may confirm it by codicil made during a lucid period. Provided a will is, on the face of it, rational and prepared in the manner required by the law it will be presumed to have been made by someone of competent testamentary capacity until proved otherwise.

Evidence

Clearly the mental state of a witness is important in assessing the value to be placed on his evidence in court. There is no general rule in this area and the court would assess the ability of each witness where any questions of his mental capacity arose. The fact that he has some sort of mental defect does not necessarily exclude his evidence. Thus, in *R v Hill 1851,* an eye witness to manslaughter by an asylum attendant was a lunatic who was grossly deluded. He believed he was attended by spirits and 20,000 of them accompanied him into the witness box. However, the court found that he was rational on other matters and understood the oath and therefore was a competent witness.

Where a court has to decide whether an individual was intoxicated either by drink or drugs the evidence of a doctor as to intoxication or sobriety is regarded as expert evidence.

Conclusion

These miscellaneous legal provisions relating to drugs, poisons, medicines and alcohol are only a small portion of the various controls that exist. Thus the measurement of the quantities of these and other substances is controlled by the Weights and Measures Act 1963 and 1979; the supply and use of radioactive materials and equipment is controlled by the Radioactive Substances Act 1948; the extent to which poisons and medicines may be given to wild animals is controlled by the Protection of Animals Act 1911, the Animals (Cruel Poisons) Act 1962 and the Protection of Birds Act 1954-67. The disposal of toxic waste and pollution of land, water or air by poisons is dealt with by the Control of Pollution Act 1974, while the provision of a safe working environment is dealt with by the Health and Safety at Work Etc Act 1974. Among other things, the Act requires an employer to conduct his business so as not to expose people to any risk to their health or safety and requires employees to take reasonable care of themselves and not to expose others to health and safety hazards. Clearly, where a toxic or potentially hazardous substance is concerned, this is particularly important.

Finally, it should be noted that already there are three EEC directives (EEC 65/65, EEC 75/319 and 320) dealing with the standardisation of controls on medicines and further European controls on all of the substances dealt with in this book may be expected over the next decade.

Further Reading

The Law Relating to the Misuse of Drugs
by P. W. H. Lydiate
Butterworth London 1977

Pharmacy Law and Ethics
by J. R. Dale and G. E. Appelbe
The Pharmaceutical Press. London 2nd Edition 1979

Law Relating to Hospitals and Kindred Institutions
by S. R. Speller
K. K. Lewis London 1978

Questions

J. S. Mill, the Utilitarian said, "The only purpose for which power can be rightfully exercised over any member of a civilised community is to prevent harm to others." To what extent has Parliament followed this dictum in legislation relating to drugs, poisons and medicines, and to what extent has it gone beyond it?

The eminent jurist Jhering defined law as a means whereby conflicting interests in society may be resolved. What conflicting interests are presented by the existence of dangerous drugs, poisons and medicinal products in any modern society, and in what way does the present English legislation upon these substances seek to achieve a balance between them?

What benefits and dangers are inherent in dangerous drugs, poisons and medicinal products? How does modern English legislation on these substances seek to minimise these dangers while preserving the benefits? To what extent do you consider this is achieved?

What do you understand by delegated legislation? How does it operate and what are its benefits and shortcomings? Illustrate your answer by reference to the Medicines Act 1968, the Dangerous Drugs Act 1971 and the Poisons Act 1972.

Give a brief historical account of the development of the law relating to dangerous drugs, poisons and medicinal products. What lessons have been learnt from this development that influence the modern legislation on these substances?

The Misuse of Drugs Act 1971 classifies dangerous drugs in two distinct ways. Outline both methods of classification and explain their significance. To what extent do you consider this dual classification satisfactory?

The Misuse of Drugs Act 1971 creates a variety of criminal offences relating to listed drugs. Give an account of these offences.

A doctor has been convicted of illegally possessing a small quantity of marihuana for smoking. Subsequent investigations suggest that he may have been overprescribing certain listed drugs for his "hippy" friends. What action may the Secretary of State for the Home Department take under the Misuse of Drugs Act 1971 in respect of this doctor?

Give an account of the activities of any *four* of the following: the Advisory Council on the Misuse of Drugs; the Poisons Board; the Medicines Commission; the Committee on Safety of Medicines; the Medicines Division of the DHSS; the British Pharmacopoeia Commission.

Outline the documentation required by the Misuse of Drugs Regulations 1973 in respect of listed drugs.

Outline the law relating to a doctor's prescription for (1) listed drugs; (2) medicinal products and (3) methylated spirits.

A doctor's freedom to prescribe whatever substance he chooses for any patient has been limited to some extent by the Misuse of Drugs Act 1971. Explain how and why.

Give a broad outline of the requirements of the Misuse of Drugs (Notification of and Supply to Addicts) Regulations 1973.

How satisfactory do you consider the legal definition of a poison? Outline the controls imposed on poisons by the Poisons Act 1972.

English Law imposes several controls on supplying poisons. Give an account of these controls.

Compare and contrast how the provisions of the Misuse of Drugs Act 1971, the Poisons Act 1972 and the Medicines Act 1968 are enforced.

What are the broad objectives of the Poisons Rules 1978? How do the rules seek to achieve these objectives?

What is a 'medicinal product' within the meaning of the Medicines Act 1968? Outline the administrative system set up by the Act to control medicinal products.

The Medicines Act 1968 adopts a licensing system to control many activities with medicinal products. State what activities are controlled by what type of licence, and give an account of the operation of the system.

Write brief notes on *four* of the following: Product Licences; the Medicines Commission; the Poisons List; Midwives and Pethidine; Delegated legislation; the Committee on Safety of Medicines; Clinical Trials in Hospitals.

What restrictions are imposed on the sale of medicinal products to the general public?

Distinguish between pharmacy only, general sales list and prescription only products. Outline the controls imposed on each category and any exemptions to these controls.

What controls are imposed on the advertising of medicinal products to (1) the medical profession and (2) the general public? What are the objectives of such controls?

What legal controls are imposed on the containers in which dangerous drugs, poisons and medicinal products may be packed? What are the related labelling requirements?

Many activities that would otherwise be unlawful under the Medicines Act 1968, the Misuse of Drugs Act 1971 and the Poisons Act 1972 may legally be carried out by a retail pharmacy business. Define such a business, and in respect of two of these Acts give an account of these activities.

Alcohol, barbiturates and tobacco are in an anomalous position as far as the controls imposed by the Medicines Act 1968, the Misuse of Drugs Act 1971 and the Poisons Act 1972 are concerned. Explain this statement and suggest reasons why this is the situation. What controls do exist on these three substances?

Outline the law concerning methylated spirits.

Write notes on *four* of the following: the licensing laws; the British Pharmacopoeia; abortion; drunken driving; the Poison Rules; prescriptions for dangerous drugs.

Give an account of the present law on abortion.

Give an account of the present law on alcohol, drugs and driving.

To what extent do you consider the present law on dangerous drugs, poisons and medicinal products provides an adequate control on these substances? Suggest ways in which the law could be improved.

Index

Ravenswood Legal Publications

Studies in Law and Practice for Health Service Management

1 **Medical Negligence**
By W. A. J. Farndale. Revised. 2nd edition.
This small volume has a series of legal case studies on claims by patients against hospital authorities based on the tort of negligence.

2 **Law on Human Transplants and Bequest of Bodies**
By W. A. J. Farndale
"A useful reference book, setting out the current legal situation in clear terms, disentangled from emotive views . . . "
Nursing Times

3 **Law on Redundancy Payments**
By W. A. J. Farndale and A. J. Cooper
"A useful book which contains details of the special redundancy provision for the National Health Service."
Industrial Law Journal

4 **Legal Liability for Claims arising from Hospital Treatment**
By W. A. J. Farndale and E. C. Larman – 2nd edition.
"Students will find this small book useful."
Solicitor Journal

5 **Legal Aspects of the Medical and Nursing Service**
By Michael H. Whincup. 2nd edition, revised and enlarged.
"Mr. Whincup possesses the enviable gift of being able to take large masses of complex and sometimes controversial doctrine and expound it in a way which means something to the layman yet does not offend the expert . . . a very valuable aid.
British Journal of Industrial Medicine

6 **Occupiers' Liability Act 1957 and the Liability of Hospitals**
By B. Williams
"One of the uniformly excellent series of Legal Case Studies, a model of clarity and conciseness."
British Journal of Industrial Medicine
"Useful and written by a legally qualified health service administrator."
The Lancet

7 **Law on Accidents to Health Service Staff and Volunteers**
By W. A. J. Farndale and Susan Russell
"The Ravenswood series of 'Law and Practice for Health Service Management' continues its practical help to managers. The rights and responsibilities of employers, employees and of volunteers are discussed in a way which is easy to understand."
Health and Social Services Journal
"This is a useful book, clearly set out and accurate enough . . . "
Health Services Manpower Review

8 **Law on Hospital Consent Forms**
By W. A. J. Farndale
This sets out the law on consent forms for operations and discusses legal, administrative and ethical principles.

9 **Law on Poisons, Medicines and Related Substances**
By P. F. C. Bayliss
An account of the legal controls on poisons, dangerous drugs and medicines by Dr. Bayliss who is qualified in medicine and law.

10 **Medico-Legal Problems in Hospital Practice**
By Dr. J. L. Brennan, M.D., Barrister

11 **Digest and Journal of Health Service Law (Issue No. 1)**
Edited by W. A. J. Farndale. Subscriptions invited.

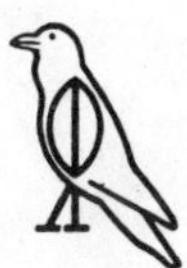

RAVENSWOOD PUBLICATIONS Ltd
P.O. Box 24, 205 Croydon Road, Beckenham, Kent, BR3 3AL, England.